CW00518642

Robson's Approach To Anatomy

by Dr David Robson, M.D., M.A.

Part I

The Skeleton

This book is dedicated to my wife,
Patricia Hamilton
whose love, support and encouragement
inspired me to write this book

ROBSON'S APPROACH TO ANATOMY

This book is part I of a seven part set. The complete set of books makes up a highly detailed, informative view of anatomy.

The complete set comprises of the books listed below:

Part I	-	The Skeleton
Part II	-	The Back
Part III	-	Head and Neck -
	-	The Nervous System
Part IV	-	The Upper Limb
Part V	-	Thorax
Part VI	-	Abdomen and Pelvis
Part VII	-	The Lower Limb

ACKNOWLEDGEMENT

I would like to thank Linda Main for her support, understanding, and all her hard work.

FOREWORD

The word anatomy is originally of Greek origin signifying dissection or cutting up; as every animal body is subject to anatomy, we divide it into human and comparative. The former is confined to the human body, the latter to the whole animal kingdom.

The book is written as a topographical or regional as opposed to a systemic textbook, the comparative will only be introduced occasionally, where it illustrates the other.

Aristotle (384 – 322 B.C.) gave the subject its scientific name, "Anatome". He was the favourite pupil of Plato (427 – 347 B.C.)

ISBN 978-0-9567521-0-9

© Copyright 2010 Dr David Robson

All illustrations and photographs are by the author.

No reproduction can be made without the express prior permission of the author.

Designed and printed by Printwell Colour Printers Ltd, Airdrie, Scotland

Published by Hamilton Publishing

INTRODUCTION

The anatomy of man can be studied from two different approaches, the morphological and the utilitarian. Students of medicine regard the human body as an apparatus liable to disorder and injury whose mechanism it behoves him to know, in order that he may be able to deal with its diseased conditions. An adequate knowledge of human anatomy can only be obtained from careful dissection. To the practitioner of medicine or surgery, such an accurate knowledge is essential, as it will enable him to place his finger over, or the point of a needle in, any required part; as well as to understand the structure of the part so indicated. Any less knowledge is of little value.

The human body consists of combination of ten systems: Skeletal, Muscular, Nervous, Digestive, Circulatory, Excretory, Reproductive, Endocrine, Respiratory and Lymphatic. Each system is made up of a set of organs; each organ is built up of tissues, who's ultimate constituents are called form elements. The names given to the various parts of the body are singularly heterogeneous. In the literature of anatomy there are over 14,800 names, many names are so linked with the history of the science that they should not be altered. Opinions differ as to the propriety of retaining the personal element in anatomical nomenclature. I have therefore retained such names wherever they constitute historical memorials of discovery; it would be a pity to divorce the names of Bell, Colles, Eustachi, Monro, Versalius or Wharton from the parts with which their names have so long been associated. Anatomy is the scientific basis of medicine and surgery, and is as important today as at any time.

HISTORICAL BACKGROUND

The earliest records of anatomical observations are those found in the writings of Alcmaeon (*fl* 470 B.C.) a native of Croton in Southern Italy. About 400 B.C. Athens became the main centre for anatomy, after Alexander's death in 323 B.C. the main centre for anatomical activity became the Egyptian city of Alexandria. The study of human anatomy dates from around 300 BC. Aristotle (384 – 322 B.C.) was one of the earliest students of the subject; he gave the science its name "Anatome" which means "cutting up". The Alexandrian school under the anatomists Herephilus (330 – 260 B.C.) and Erasistratus (330 – 255 B.C.) became the chief centre of anatomical study in the world.

In the second century A.D. Galen (130 – 200 A.D.) contributed significantly to the study of anatomy, his voluminous works included seven on anatomy. Henri de Mondeville (1260 – 1320) of Montpellier in the late thirteenth century was the first person who is known to have lectured from illustrations. Mondino de Luzzi (c. 1270 – 1326) carried our the first recorded human dissection in Bologna around 1315, his Anatomia Mundini (1316) became the standard text on the subject. The first printed version appeared in 1478. Modern anatomy begins in the sixteenth century when Andreas Vesalius (1514 – 1563) professor of anatomy at Padua published his great masterpiece, the De Humani Corporis Fabrica, in 1543. Gabriele Falloppia (1523 – 1563) succeeded Vesalius at Padua, he published his Observationes Anatomicae in (1561). The greatest comparative anatomist was one of Fallopia's pupils, Hieronymus Fabricus ab Aquapendente (Fabrizio c. 1533 – 1619) his most significant work was De Venarum Ostiolis (1603). This work was to prove an inspiration to William Harvey (1578 – 1657). Anatomy became integrated into learned medicine in England thanks to John Caius (1510 – 1573). The first printed textbook in English, The Anatomie of the Body of Man by Thomas Vicary (1490 – 1561) was published in (1548). The sixteenth century had revealed that the structures of the body were not as Galen has stated, and that dissection was revealing structures unknown to the earlier anatomists. In England in the seventeenth century, Thomas Willis (1621 – 1675) pioneered the study of the brain and nervous system, discovering the Circulus Arteriosus at the base of the brain in (1664). In the eighteenth century research into general anatomy continued along the lines of Vesalius and his followers. In 1768 William Hunter (1718 – 1783) opened his Windmill Street School which by the 1770's had become one of the most famous anatomy schools in the world. He was a great anatomist and obstetrician and published his book Anatomia Uteri Humani Gravidi (1774).

His brother John, (1728 – 1793) was the first to apply the results of research to anatomy and surgery, and is regarded as the founder of scientific surgery. In the nineteenth century knowledge of human anatomy was well established. Henry Gray (1827 – 1861) published his textbook "Gray's Anatomy" in (1858). This classic is the world's oldest textbook of anatomy still in print today. Alexander Macalister (1844 – 1919) who knew more about the anatomy of the human body than any man living published his great textbook of anatomy in 1889. He held the chair of anatomy at Cambridge for thirty six years, the same length of time as Sir William Turner held the corresponding chair at Edinburgh. In the twentieth century anatomy is taught in relation to clinical medicine and surgery.

DESCRIPTIVE TERMS

In anatomical description the body is supposed to stand upright, so that the upwards means respectively towards the head (cranial) and downwards means respectively towards the feet (distal). The anterior surface of the body is called ventral and the posterior dorsal. The aspect of any part near to, or directed towards the head is called proximal, while that directed from the head is distal. The terms superficial and deep are applied to parts according as they nearer to, or farther from the skin. Pre and post axial indicate aspect rather than position. A vertical plane or section carried from before backwards is called a sagittal section, while a section in the vertical plane at right angles to this is said to be coronal. Thus a skull divided vertically from nose to nape, into lateral portions is sagittally divided; but if cut vertically from ear to ear and so divided into fore and hind halves, the section is "coronal".

The sagittal plane which divides the body into symmetrical lateral halves is the median plane, which intersects the surface before and behind in the anterior and posterior median lines. According to their relation to this plane, parts are divided into medial (nearer, or directed towards the median plane), and lateral (or farther away on each side of it). Thus that aspect of a limb which is directed towards the median plane is the "medial aspect" and the opposite is the "lateral". There are also horizontal planes which traverse the body at right angles to both the median and coronal planes.

VARIABILITY

No two human bodies are exactly alike in the details of organisation. Inheritance, habitual action, occupation and other circumstances of environment are factors which act with unequal intensity in the history of each individual, modifying the proportional development of parts. Although the resulting range of variety is great, yet there are certain conditions of each part which, from their frequency of occurrence it is convenient to call normal. These anomalies may be grouped into the following categories:

1. **Embryonal** – The persistence in the adult of conditions usually transient in the foetus. 2. **Atavistic** – The occurrence of conditions which existed in ancestral forms, but which have disappeared even from human foetus, under the action of environing influences. These two groups are closely related.

3. **Retrogressive** – Due to lack of nourishment of parts causing their atrophy, degeneration or disappearance; loss of function having proceeded degeneration of structure. 4. **Vicarious** - Alterations due to the assumption of supplementary functions by certain parts, compensating for the deficiencies of others. 5. **Progressive** - Due to increasing function and foreshadowing increase of specialisation.

CONTENTS

"THE SKELETON"

Historical Background
Osteology
Classification of Bones
Sesamoid Bones
Articulations
Vertebrae
Cervical
Atlas and Axis
The Seventh Cervical
Thoracic Vertebrae
Lumbar Vertebrae
Table of the Characteristics of the Vertebrae
Trabecular Arrangement of Vertebrae
The Sacrum
The Coccyx
Sternum and Ribs
The Ribs
The Thorax
The Appendicular Skeleton
The Clavicle
The Scapula
The Humerus
The Radius
The Ulna

The Hand - a) Carpals b) Metacarpals c) Phalanges

The Hip Bone
The Pelvis
The Femur
The Patella
The Tibia
The Fibula

The Foot - a) The Tarsals b) Metatarsals c) Phalanges

CONTENTS - Continued

"THE SKULL"

The Skull at Birth
Epipteric Bones
Wormian Bones
The Frontal Bone
The Parietal Bones
The Occipital Bones
The Sphenoid Bone
The Temporal Bone
The Tympanic Bone
The Petrous Bone
The Ethmoid Bone
The Vomer
The Palatine Bone
The Nasal Bones
The Lacrimal Bones
The Zygomatic Bone
The Maxilla
The Mandible
The Hyoid Bone
The Auditory Ossicles
The Skull as a Whole
The Exterior of the Skull
The Interior of the Skull
The Interior of the Cranium
The Foramina of the Skull

Medical Personalities

Bibliography

OSTEOLOGY

The general framework of the human body is built-up of a series of bones supplemented in certain regions by pieces of cartilage; this bony and cartilaginous framework constitutes the skeleton.

In many animals the skeleton consists of an inner or deep skeleton, which is called endoskeleton, and an external or superficial the exoskeleton. In the case of the lobster or snail, they have only the exoskeleton. In the human subject the exoskeleton is very rudimentary, its only important representative being the nails and the enamel of the teeth, and therefore in human anatomy the term skeleton is confined to the endoskeleton, this is divisible into an axial part and appendicular part. The skeleton plays an indispensable role in movement by providing a strong, stable but mobile framework on which the muscles can act. It consists of a series of independently moveable levers on which the muscles can pull to move different parts of the body. The skeleton also supports and protects the body's essential organs, notably the brain which is encased in the skull, and the spinal cord in the neural canal of the vertebral column. The heart and lungs which are protected by the ribs. The ribs also make breathing possible by supporting the chest cavity so that the lungs are not compressed and by helping in the breathing movements themselves.

The skeleton is not and inert frame, it is an active organ that produces red blood cells (formed in bone marrow) it also acts a reservoir for minerals such as calcium, which can be drawn on if required by other parts of the body.

The skeleton is of mesodermal origin and in the adult consists of 206 bones, united by cartilages and ligaments. These may be conveniently arranged in two series.

1. Bones of the axial skeleton.

   A. Of the head.

a)	Cranium	8
b)	Face	14
c)	Auditory ossicles	6
d)	Hyoid bone	1
		—
		29

   B. Of the trunk

e)	Vertebral column	26
f)	Ribs	24
g)	Sternum	1
		—
		80

2. Bones of the appendicular skeleton.

h)	Shoulder girdles	4
i)	Arms and forearms	6
j)	Hands	54
k)	Pelvic girdle	2
l)	Thigh and lower leg	6
m)	Patellae	2
n)	Feet	52
		—
		206

CLASSIFICATION OF BONES

The bones of the human skeleton can be divided into several classes.

1) **Long Bones**, which are found in the limbs where they form levers; as in the lower limb sustaining the weight of the trunk and providing the means of locomotion. 2) **Flat bones**, which confer protection, or provide broad surfaces for muscular attachment, as in the case of the skull and the scapulae. 3) **Short bones**, are those bones of the skeleton that are intended for strength and compactness, and where there is limited movement as in the case of the carpus and tarsus. 4) **Pneumatic bones**, such as those found in the skull, the intervening spongy substance is called the Diploe, and this in certain regions of the skull, they undergo absorption, and air-filled spaces called sinuses are left between the tables of the skull; such bones are called pneumatic. 5) **Irregular bones** have complex shapes, such as the vertebrae, sacrum, coccyx and certain skull bones. There are additional types of bones that are not included in this classification by shape. a) **Sutural or Wormian bones**, these are small bones found between the joints of certain bones of the skull, i.e., in the Lamboid suture separating parietal from occipital. b) **Epipteric bones**, these are scale-like bones which occupy the antero-lateral fontanelles. c) **Sesamoid bones**, these are small bones found in the tendon of certain muscles. Long bones have hollow shafts (diaphyses), and articular extremities, which ossify independently of the shafts, and which, before their union therewith, are called epiphyses.

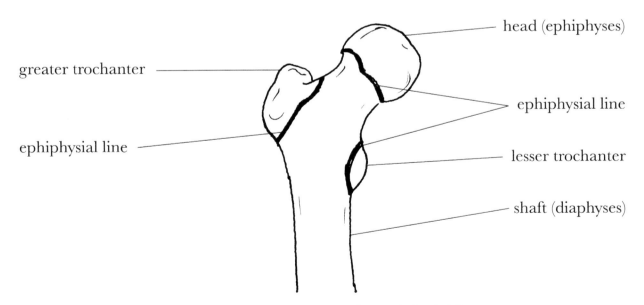

Upper end right femur, showing epiphysial lines.

Epiphyses; may be divided under three headings, 1) Those which appear at the articular ends of bones as in the lower limb where there is a transmission of weight from one bone to another, these are termed pressure epiphysis. 2) Traction epiphyses; example the greater and lesser trochanter, where there is inserted a number of muscles. Traction epiphyses, originally sesamoid structures though not necessarily sesamoid bones. 3) Atavistic epiphyses, are those representing parts of the skeleton which at one time formed separate bones; but which only appear as separate ossifications in early life, example the skull.

SESAMOID BONES

Sesamoid bones are small rounded masses which are cartilaginous in early life, but become osseous in the adult. They are developed in tendons where they exert a certain amount of pressure upon the parts they glide over; there are two types. a) Those that are found in tendons. b) Those that are related to the articular ends of certain bones; the latter in relation to the head of the first metatarsal are weight bearing. The former of which the patella is the largest, is found in the front of the knee joint in the back of the quadriceps tendon. Associated with the lateral head of gastrocnemius is a sesamoid bone known as the fabella, sesamoid bones are also found in the tendon of peroneus longus, tibialis anterior, in the tendon iliopsoas, gluteus maximus, and occasionally in the tendon of biceps just before its insertion into bicipital tuberosity of the radius.

THE SURFACE OF BONES

The surface of bones presents for study: 1) articular extremities whose shapes depend on the direction and amount of the movements in the joints which they form. 2) surfaces, sculptured in relief by their relation to soft parts, here and there raised into round blunt eminences, or obtuse knobs (tubercles), or sharper points (spines), or lines or crests, or other irregularities which are known by the generic name of processes. In other places bones are depressed into fossae or sulci, which are either real hollows made by the pressure of some contiguous part, or apparent grooves left by the elevation above the original surface of two marginal ridges. Perforations in bone may be either for the transmission of vessels or nerves, or else spaces of deficient ossification.

ARTICULATIONS

The place where two bones come into contact with each other is called a joint or articulation, in the simplest form of which the contiguous ends are fastened together by an intervening mass of connective tissue. Joints of this class are called **Synarthroses**, and they differ among themselves according to the nature of the uniting medium, the shapes of the opposed surfaces and the widths of the intervals between the bones. The immovable articulations of the contiguous margins of flat bones with a minimum of intervening tissue is a **suture**, which if the edges be even and evenly applied is harmonic, as illustrated by the joints around the nasal bone.

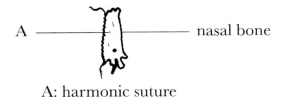

A: harmonic suture

If one margin overlap the other, it is a squamous suture; if the edges be toothed, and interlock, with teeth tapering points, it is serrate; if they dovetail, it is dentate; should the interlocking edges alternately overlap, it is a limbous suture.

The tempro-parietal joint between the temporal (c) and the parietal (d), is an example of a squamous suture;

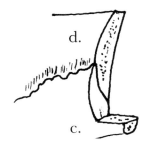

The inter-parietal of a serrate (d); the occipito-parietal (c) of a dentate; and the fronto-parietal of a limbous suture as the frontal (e) overlaps the parietal (f).

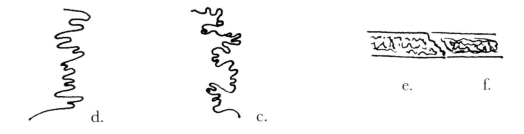

When a ridge of one bone is received into a groove of another, the joint is called a **Schindylesis**, as in the union of the vomer with the sphenoid; and if a peg of one bone be received into a mortice in another, as the teeth in their sockets, the joint is called **Gomphosis**. When the interval between the bones is wider, so that the uniting connective tissue is elongated into ligamentous bands, the joint is called **Syndesmosis**; and if the ligament be flattened into a thin expansion, it is called an interosseous membrane. When the connecting substance is cartilage, the joint is called **Synchondrosis**, and such joints may be of two types; true, when they arise by the formation of two separate and approaching ossifications in a continuous cartilage, such as the joint between each epyphysis and diaphysis in a long bone; or false, when the tissue is fibro-cartilage, not hyaline, formed by the chondrification of the medium uniting two originally separate bones, as in the sacro-iliac or inter-pubic joints. None of the bony surfaces of these joints have an investing periosteum. In the majority of joints, the contiguous surfaces are not separated by intervening tissue, but are in contact with each other, forming opposite sides of a free space (the cavity of the joint). These surfaces remain cartilaginous, naked, and smooth, and the layer of fibrous tissue which invests the cavity circumferentially, and which is continuous on each side with the periosteum of the component bones, is called the **Capsular ligament**. The inner surface of this is imperfectly lined with a layer of flattened endothelial cella, which with the inner capsule, constitutes **Synovial membrane**, and covers the lateral walls of the cavity of the joint, except such parts as encrusted with articular (hyaline) cartilage. These moveable joints with a cavity are called **Diathroses**.

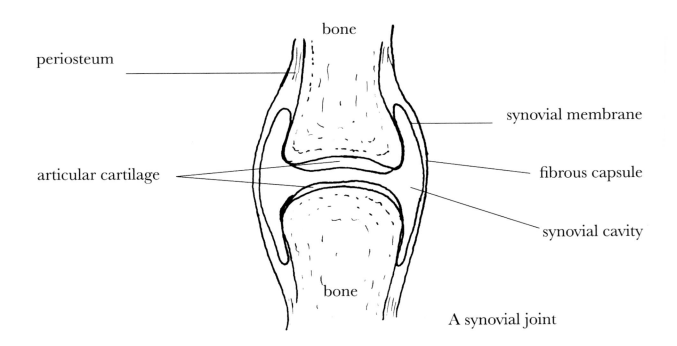

A synovial joint

The cartilage surfaces are remarkably smooth; the coefficient of friction of cartilage upon cartilage when moistened by synovial being exceedingly small. Synovial fluid is an exudation containing mucin, formed on the surfaces of the villi and folds which fringe the margins of reflections of synovial membranes. The size of the cavity of each joint is invariable, and is correlated with the extent of it mobility. In some very moveable joints, such as the hip and elbow, where certain positions are larger and in others are lesser, bulk of one bone is received into a cavity in the other, masses of fat are disposed outside the synovial membrane and inside the capsular ligament; so that in the latter case they are made to bulge into the joint by the tension of the overlying ligament, while in the former they are pushed out into extra-articular recesses. Such masses of fat are called **Haversian glands**.

Havers, C. (1657 – 1702)

VERTEBRAE

The human vertebral column consists of thirty-three vertebrae; the upper twenty-four are called true as they remain separate during life; while the lower nine are called false; because they become consolidated into two masses. The lower four or caudal vertebrae, are rudimentary and ankylose together to form the coccyx, and the five above these unite to form the sacrum. The seven uppermost true vertebrae are called cervical and make the skeleton of the neck; the topmost or atlas articulating with the occipital condyles of the base of the skull; the twelve succeeding are thoracic and bare moveable ribs; the five remaining are called lumbar, the lowest of which articulates with the sacrum. Each vertebrae consists of a body, arch and process, the body is a disc of cancellous bone, whose upper and lower surfaces are joined to its predecessor and successor by a soft intervertebral fibro-cartilage, so that the whole series builds up a flexible column of support for the trunk. Each body is transversely convex and vertically concave anteriorly, but flat or transversely concave posteriorly, where it is pierced by one of two large foramen for the exit of vertebral veins. The arch which consists chiefly of compact bone is attached to the dorsal surface of each body, and bounds the neural canal. The whole chain of arches with their intervening ligaments makes, with the backs of the bodies the wall of the neural canal which contains the spinal cord.

Functions of the vertebral column

The vertebral column has a three fold function. First it is the strong walled canal protecting a nerve centre; second it is the basis from which the trunk muscles act; third it is the pillar of support bearing on its summit the head, laterally the arms, and anteriorly the viscera. Its length measured along its axis varies little, in the adult male it is 70cm in length, its cervical part is approximately 12cm, thoracic 28cm, lumbar 18cm, and sacrum and coccyx 12cm. In the female its total length is about 60cm.

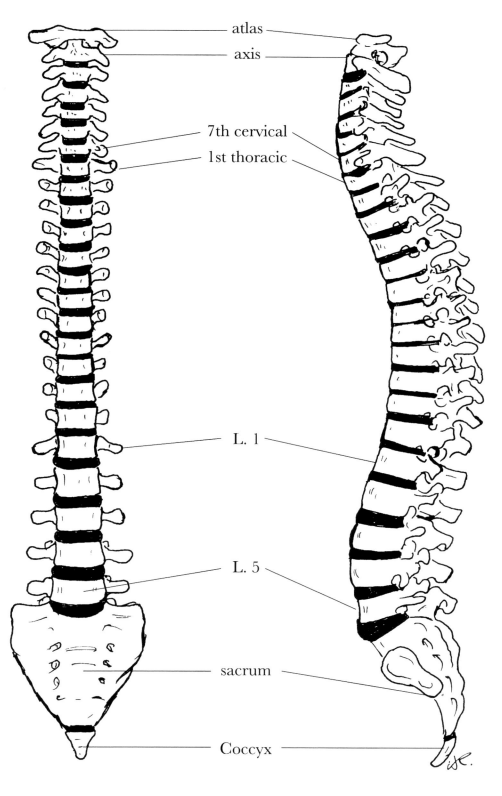

atlas

axis

7th cervical

1st thoracic

L. 1

L. 5

sacrum

Coccyx

anterior view

lateral view
showing the cervical thoracic
and lumbar curvatures.

The Vertebral Colum

The area of the canal varies at different levels, being the greatest in the regions of greatest mobility as can be seen be the following table.

Fig. 1

At the 2nd cervical it is 380 sq. mm.

At the 7th cervical it is 290 sq. mm.

At the 2nd thoracic it is 115 sq. mm.

At the 6th thoracic it is 230 sq. mm.

At the 5th lumbar it is 320 sq. mm.

At the 3rd sacral it is 80 sq. mm.

From the convex surface of the arch nine processes project, where five are for the attachment of muscles and ligaments, and four for the purpose of articulations, of the former the spinous process is singler projecting posteriorly towards the surface in the midline.

Two transverse processes for muscular attachments arise from the arch on each side and project laterally. Internal to these the arch thickens into an articular mass, from which four articular processes project, two superiorly and two inferiorly to join correlative processes of the neighbouring vertebrae. The part of the arch between the spine and articular processes, on each side, is flat rough edged and is called the lamina, while that between the articular process and the body is rounded, grooved above and below and is called the pedicle. The spaces between the successive pedicles below, are called intervertebral foramen, through which the spinal nerves emerge and the lateral spinal arteries enter the neural canal. At the root of the lamina posterior to the articular processes, there is usually a rough area for muscular attachment, which when well defined is call a tuberosity. To the side of the body, close to the base of the pedicle of each vertebrae, a costal process is appended on each side, these are small and continuously ossified into the vertebrae except in the thoracic region, where they are long and become early segmented off, forming the ribs. Each vertebrae thus consists of sixteen parts – a body, two pedicles, two lamina, a spinous process, two transverse processes, four articular processes, two tuberosities, and two costal processes.

CERVICAL VERTEBRAE

The cervical vertebrae are seven in number and are readily distinguished from the thoracic or lumbar vertebrae by the presence of a foramen in the transverse process. Although the cervical vertebrae are the smallest and densest they have the widest neural canal.

ATLAS AND AXIS

The first and second cervical vertebrae are modified to allow the head to move freely as is consistent with the safety of the spinal cord. The atlas presents above two lateral concavities with which the occipital condyles articulate, permitting a nodding motion of the head. The atlas can rotate in a horizontal plane on the axis as upon a pivot, carry the head with it.

The atlas is reduced to a ring of two arches, and two lateral masses, and its body has become separated from its anterior arch and ankolysed to the summit of the body of the axis to form the odontoid process. It is the widest transversely of the cervical vertebrae. Its anterior arch which is one-fifth of the entire ring, is vertically flattened, presenting anteriorly a tubercle, and posteriorly a concave articular facet for the odontoid process which lies posteriorly. The posterior arch is thinner, but twice as long as the anterior and forms an even parabolic curve undivided into pedicles and lamina. It bears no spinous process as any such projection would interfere with its rotation on the axis; but it has instead a rough posterior tubercle. The superior surface of this arch is grooved on each side where it joins the articular mass (sinus atlantis), for the third stage of the vertebral artery. Each lateral mass presents on its superior surface an irregular articular hollow, diverging posteriorly from its fellow, with a sharp raised outer edge, to receive the occipital condyles. Facing the neural canal on its inner side is an internal tuberosity giving attachment to the transverse ligament, which divides the hollow of the ring into two parts – a smaller anterior for the odontoid process, a larger posterior for the spinal cord. The atlas has no articular process comparable with those of other vertebrae, as the grooves for the spinal nerves lies posterior to the lateral mass. Each transverse process starts from the root of the posterior arch, close to the back of the lateral mass, and passes forwards and outwards, jutting out farther than that of any other cervical vertebrae, and ending in an obliquely placed tubercle. The costal process is shorter with a rudimentary tubercle. The internal tuberosity is divided into two parts, an anterior on the base of the costal process to which the transverse ligament is attached and posterior; between these, a branch of the vertebral artery and vein enter the bone. The long transverse process gives leverage to the rotator muscles attached to it, and lies inferiorly to the mastoid process. The suboccipital nerve lies in the sinus atlantis, medial to the artery, its anterior branch passing over the front of the costal process. The inferior articular surface like the superior is preneural and in series with the costo-vertebral joints, it is slightly concave.

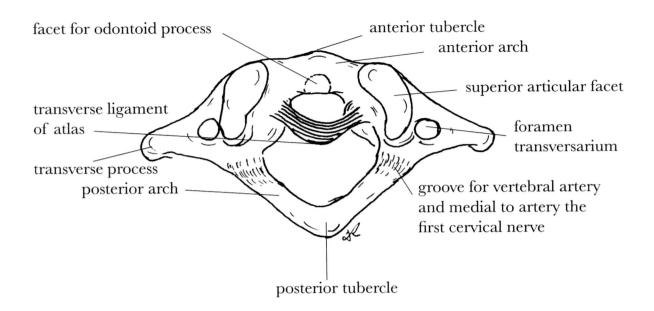

facet for odontoid process

anterior tubercle

anterior arch

superior articular facet

transverse ligament of atlas

foramen transversarium

transverse process

posterior arch

groove for vertebral artery and medial to artery the first cervical nerve

posterior tubercle

The atlas, superior aspect.

The axis is the thickest and strongest of the vertebrae of this region, and bears the ankylosed body of the atlas as the odontoid process. This articulates anteriorly with the anterior arch of the atlas behind with transverse ligament, which prevents it from pressing on the spinal cord. The superior articular processes are preneural, the inferior resemble those of the succeeding vertebrae, but are directed a little outwards as well as forwards and downwards. The costal process is thick at its base, but has a rudimental tuberosity, and the transverse process starts between the superior and inferior articular processes. The spinous process is strong with a prominent median ridge, but with depressed and short lateral tubercles. The tip of the dontoid process is pointed for the apical ligament, below this it is laterally flattened into an oblique surface on each side for the occipito-odontoid process. The lamina are stronger than those of any other cervical vertebrae.

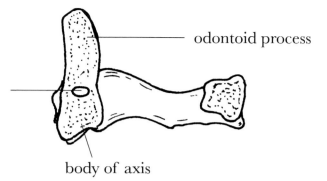

cartilage representing the intervertebral disc between the odontoid process and body of the axis.

odontoid process

body of axis

The atlas gives attachment to the following muscles:

i) Anterior arch – Longus colli.

ii) Posterior arch – Rectus capitis posterior minor.

iii) Transverse process – Rectus capitis anterior minor, rectus capitus lateralis, oblique capitis inferior, oblique capitis superior, splenius cervicis, levator scapulae and intertransversus anterior and posterior.

The axis

i) The body – Longus colli.

ii) Spinous process – Oblique capitis inferior, rectus capitis posterior major, semispinalis cervicis, interspinalis, multifidus.

iii) Transverse process – Splenius cervicis, intertransversus anterior and posterior, levator scapulae, longissimus cervicis and scalenus medius.

The seventh cervical

i) The body – Longus colli.

ii) Spinous process – Trapezius, rhomboid minor, serratus posterior superior, splenius capitis, multifidus, interspinalis, semispinalis thoracis

iii) Transverse process – Intertransversus anterior and posterior, levator costae, scalenus posterior, iliocostalis thoracis, scalenus medius, semispinalis capitis.

iv) Atricular process – Multifidus, longissimus capitis.

The seventh cervical

The seventh cervical is known as the vertebrae prominens, and has the longest spine which is easily felt at the nape of the neck. The costotransverse foramen is very small, with a weak costal process generally showing a rudimental tubercle, and giving attachment to muscles. In rare cases it is larger and segmented off forming a cervical rib. A cervical rib is less common and is present in 0.5% - 1% of people. It is the enlarged costal element of the seventh cervical vertebrae, it may be large and palpable or only detectable by a radiograph. It may be unilateral or bilateral asymptomatic or through pressure on the lower trunk of the brachial plexus or subclavian vessels produce neurovascular symptoms.

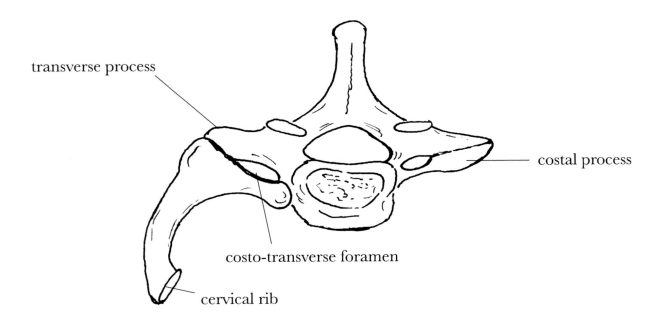

transverse process

costal process

costo-transverse foramen

cervical rib

Seventh cervical vertebra and cervical rib

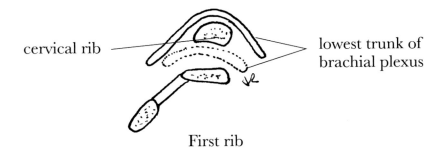

cervical rib

lowest trunk of brachial plexus

First rib

To show how a cervical rib may cause traction on the lowest trunk of the brachial plexus by angulating it, dotted line shows normal position of the trunk.

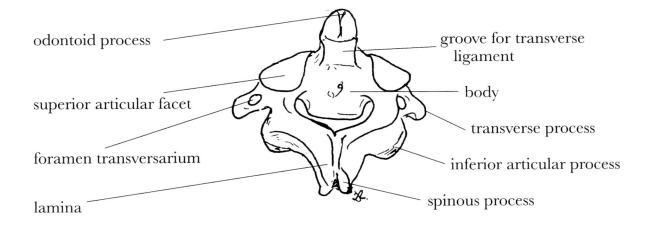

odontoid process

groove for transverse ligament

superior articular facet

body

foramen transversarium

transverse process

inferior articular process

lamina

spinous process

The axis. Posterosuperior aspect

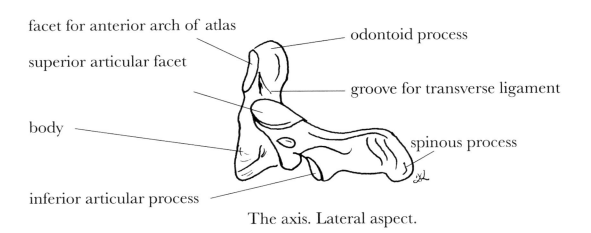

facet for anterior arch of atlas

odontoid process

superior articular facet

groove for transverse ligament

body

spinous process

inferior articular process

The axis. Lateral aspect.

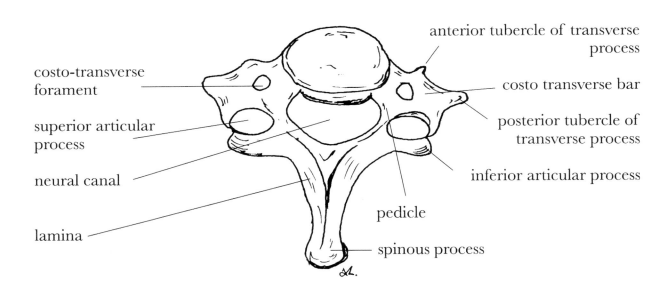

anterior tubercle of transverse process

costo-transverse forament

costo transverse bar

superior articular process

posterior tubercle of transverse process

neural canal

inferior articular process

pedicle

lamina

spinous process

The seventh cervical vertebra.

* Chassaignac pointed out that the common carotid artery can be compressed against the anterior tubercle of the transverse process of the sixth vertebrae; and is therefore named tuberculum caroticum or Chassaignac's tubercle; it also constitutes an important guide to the vertebral artery.

THORACIC VERTEBRAE

The thoracic vertebrae are twelve in number and increase successfully in size from above downwards. All are distinguished by the presence of cartilage-clad facets on the sides of the bodies, and all but the lowest two by circular facets on the transverse processes; the former articulating with the head of the rib, the latter with the tubercles of the ribs. * A typical thoracic vertebrae has a decurrrent triquetrous spinous process and has a circular neural canal.

* In quadrupeds the majority of the spinous processes of the thoracic vertebrae project upwards and backwards, while those in the lumbar region are directed upwards and forwards. The change in inclination is effected on one of the lower thoracic vertebrae, the spine of which points almost directly upwards. This vertebrae is known as the anticlinal, and in man its representative is the eleventh thoracic.

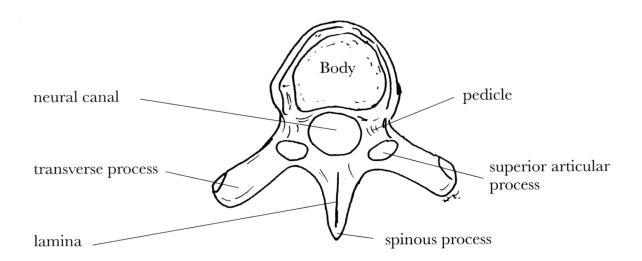

neural canal

pedicle

transverse process

superior articular process

lamina

spinous process

Body

Typical thoracic vertebra, superior aspect

* **Chassaignac**, Charles M.E. (1804 – 1879).
Tubercle of Chaissaignac, discovered 1834. Professor of Anatomy and Surgery, Paris.

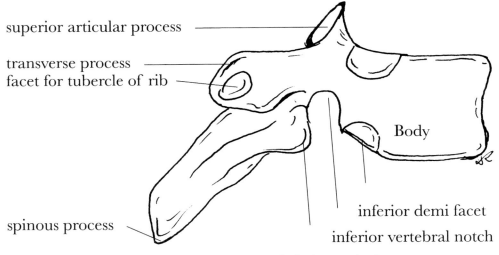

superior articular process ————————

transverse process ————————
facet for tubercle of rib ————————

Body

spinous process ————————

inferior demi facet
inferior vertebral notch
inferior articular process
Typical thoracic vertebra, lateral aspect.

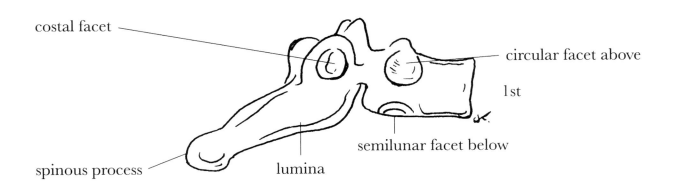

costal facet ————————

circular facet above

1st

spinous process ————————   lumina

semilunar facet below

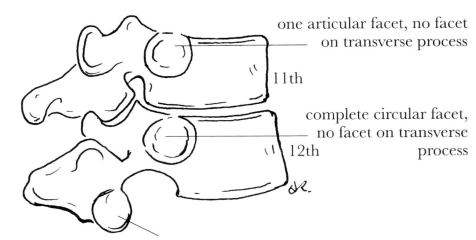

one articular facet, no facet
on transverse process

11th

complete circular facet,
no facet on transverse
12th   process

Inferior articular process convex and turned lateralwards

First, Eleventh and Twelfth Thracic vertebrae

LUMBAR VERTEBRAE

The lumbar vertebrae are five in number and are the largest of the moveable vertebrae, they are distinguished by the absence of the foramen in their transverse processes, and of a costal facet on the sides of the bodies, they exhibit a triangular neural canal.

The fifth lumbar is characterised by its body being considerably deeper in front than behind, this is a condition which accords with the prominence of the sacrovertebral articulation. By the small size of its spinous process; by the wide interval between the inferior articular processes; and by the thickness of its transverse processes which spring from the body as well as from the pedicles.

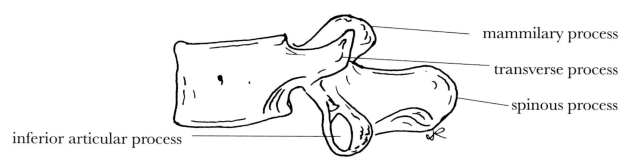

mammilary process

transverse process

spinous process

inferior articular process

Fourth lumbar vertebra, lateral aspect

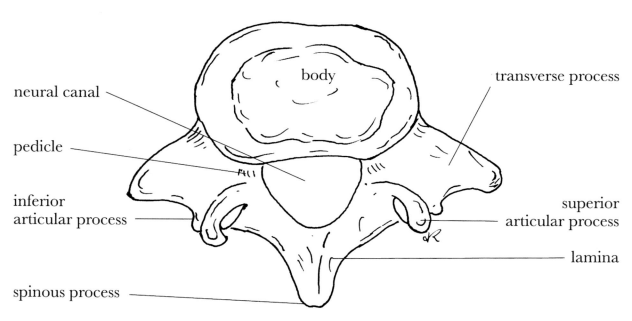

body

transverse process

neural canal

pedicle

inferior
articular process

superior
articular process

lamina

spinous process

Fifth lumbar vertebra, superior aspect

The following table exhibits the characteristics of the vertebrae from each region

	CERVICAL	THORACIC	LUMBAR
BODIES	Broadest transversely surfaces concave, No costal facets.	Nearly equal transversely and sagitally Surfaces flat, costal facets.	Broadest transversely surfaces flat. No costal facets.
PEDICLES	With neuro-central lips lateral, and Sagitally placed, notched above and Below.	Neuro-central lips rudimental, posterior Transversely placed, notched below.	No neuro-central lips, deeply notched Below.
LAMINA SPINES	Long, thin and flattened. Bifid, depressed with weak median ridge And diverging lateral tubercles.	Short, Vertically elongated. Long, decurrent imbricating with single terminal tubercle and strong median ridge.	Short, rough vertically elongated. Quadrate, directed backwards horizontally reduced to median ridge.
COSTAL PROCESSES	Flat- slender, continuously ossified to vertebrae, forming front boundary of foramen.	A detached bone (Rib).	Continuously ossified to vertebra, flat and thin.
TRANSVERSE PROCESSES	Directed forwards forming outer boundary of foramen — joined to costal process by bony lamella.	Directed backwards articulating with rib by ligaments.	A rudimental spur (accessory process).
TUBEROSITIES	Sessile on back of inferior articular process.	On back of transverse process and inseparable from it.	A protuberance outside the upper articular process. (Mammillary process).
SPINAL FORAMEN	Triangular, elongated transversely.	Circular.	Triangular elongated transversely.
UPPER ARTICULAR PROCESSES	Flat, directed backwards and superiorly.	Flat, backwards and outwards.	Concave transversely backwards and inwards.
LOWER ARTICULAR PROCESSES	Flat, directed forwards and inferiorly. Axes of articular surfaces slightly converge downwards and forwards.	Flat, forwards and inwards. Cut edges of articular surfaces horizontally divided coincide with arcs of a circle whose centre is situated at anterior lip of body in mid-line.	Convex, forwards and outwards. Cut edges of articular surfaces horizontally divided coincide with arcs of a circle whose centre is at the root of the spinous process.

TRABECULAR ARRANGEMENT OF VERTEBRAE

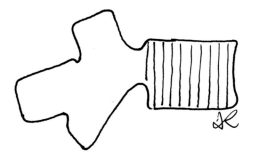

Vertical trabeculae mainly support the body and the compressive forces help to sustain the body weight.

A.

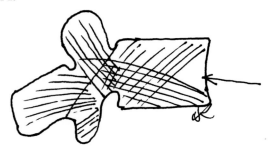

Inferior and superior oblique patterns.

NB. Segment of relative weakness.

B.

The other trabecular system helps to resist shearing forces at both the lower and upper surfaces of the body there are oblique trabeculae, which aid in compressive load bearing function and also serve to resist the bending and tensile forces that occur at the pedicles and spinous processes Figs. B &C.

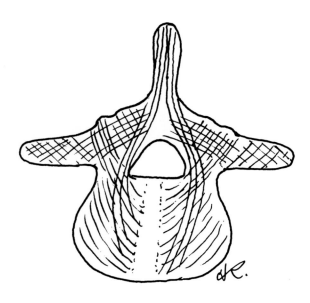

C.

Oblique patterns viewed from above.

THE SACRUM

The sacrum is a large, wedge shaped bone which is formed by the fusion of the five sacral vertebra. The sacrum is situated at the upper and posterior part of the pelvic cavity, where it is inserted like a wedge between the two innominate bones. Its base projects upwards and forwards to articulate with the fifth lumbar vertebra to form the prominent sacro-vertebral angle; its apex articulates with the coccyx. It has a pelvic, a dorsal, two lateral surfaces, abase, an apex, and a central canal.

The first sacral represents the sixth lumbar vertebra of most quadrupeds, which has become assimilated owing to the upward growth of the pelvic bones correlated with the upright position, this should be taken into account in comparing the numerical relations of the human vertebra with those of mammals. The fourth and fifth sacral vertebrae represent the first and second caudal vertebrae of mammals. The two true sacral vertebrae being the second and third. The varying conditions of the lumbosacral region especially in the lower races of man depend on these changes. The sacrum bears the weight of the upper part of the body and transmits it to the ilia which rests on the thighs. The method of transmission is two-fold, the bone from its shape serves as a key-stone for the pelvic arch; while on the other hand, even when the articular surfaces are partly chiselled away, the bone is so firmly slung by the strong posterior sacro-iliac ligaments that the fixity of the pelvic arch is preserved. The ala in consequence have a very hard shell of compact tissue, and the transverse or traction planes of the cancelli are thick and definite, though the cancellous meshes are wide especially below.

The sacrum as a whole articulates with four bones, the two inominate bones, coccyx, and the fifth lumbar vertebra. It gives origin to five pairs of muscles and twenty ligaments.

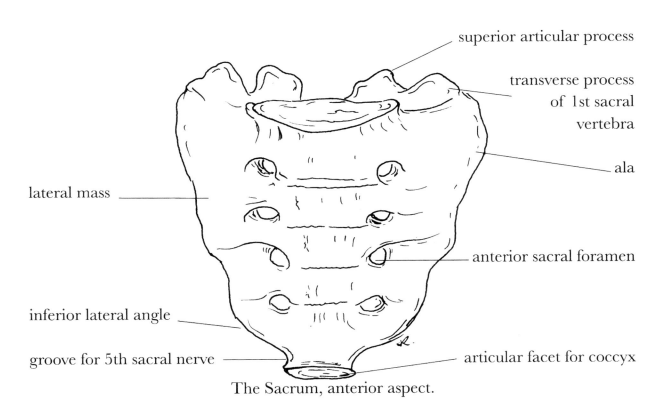

The Sacrum, anterior aspect.

THE COCCYX

The caudal vertebrae are represented by rudimental bodies without arches, which in the adult ultimately fuse into a single bone. The first piece is transversely elongated with an elliptical upper facet united by fibro-cartilage to the fifth sacral vertebrae having a small rudimentary transverse process projecting out from each side, and a cornu or pedicle projecting upwards and united by fibrous tissue to the cornu of the sacrum. In the second vertebrae these are represented by two little tubercles, the third is an irregular bony nodule, and the fourth is still more irregular being an ossification, not in one vertebral body but in a fibro-cartilaginous knob formed by the union of the rudimental bodies of the four hindmost vertebrae of the human tail.

The coccyx as a whole is triangular, concave anteriorly continuing the curve of the sacrum, crossed by three lines of intervertebral ankylosis; the posterior surface is convex and the edges rough, presenting three notches. The apex is generally nodose.

The coccyx is composed of four vertebrae, but the number may be increased to five or reduced to three. It articulates with only the sacrum, and gives attachment to three pairs of muscles and three pairs of ligaments.

Ossification of the sacrum resembles that of a typical vertebrae. Primary centres for the centrum and each half of the vertebral arch appear between the tenth and twentieth weeks. The primary centres for the costal elements of the upper three or more sacral vertebrae appear above and lateral to the pelvic sacral foramina, between the sixth and eighth months of intrauterine life.

The Coccyx

Each segment of the coccyx is ossified from one primary centre. The centre for the first segment appears at birth. The remaining segments ossify at varying intervals up to the twentieth year.

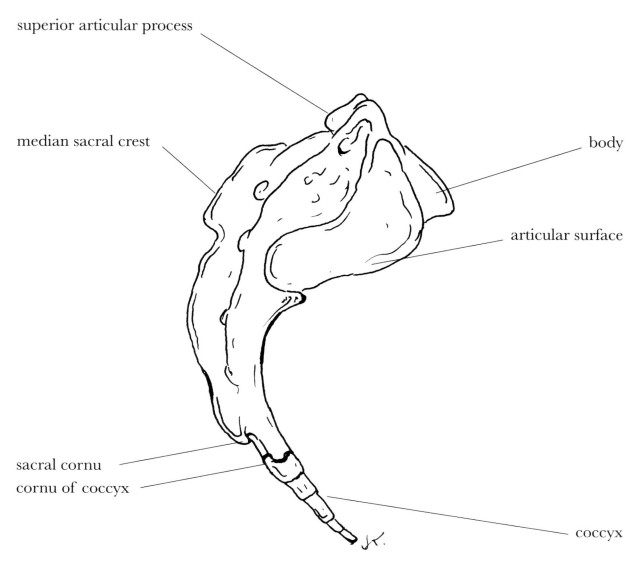

superior articular process

median sacral crest

body

articular surface

sacral cornu

cornu of coccyx

coccyx

Sacrum and coccyx, right lateral aspect.

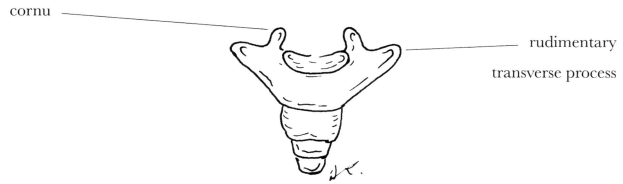

cornu

rudimentary

transverse process

The coccyx, anterior aspect.

STERNUM AND RIBS

The sternum is an oblong, flat, spongy bone situated in the middle portion of the anterior wall of the thorax. It consists of three parts (a) the manubrium sterni (presternum), (b) the gladiolus (mesosternum), constituting the body, (c) the xiphoid or ensiform process (metasternum). It originally consisted of six segments of which four have fused to form the body. The manubrium is a triangular broad bone, with four borders, a broad one above processing a suprasternal notch, an articular surface below for the body of the sternum, and two lateral sloping edges marked from above, downwards by three areas, i.e. an oval saddle – shaped facet for the medial end of the clavicle, an impression for the first costal cartilage and at the lower angle a demi-facet for the second costal cartilage. The anterior aspect of the junction of the manubrium and body forms the sternal angle and an important landmark in surface topography as it gives the location of the second costal cartilage and rib. The joint between the manubrium and body is called the manubrosternal junction or angle of Louis. This joint allows slight movement between the manubrium and body, when the ribs rise and fall during breathing.

Louis, P.C.A. (1787-1872)

The anterior surface of the body is convex and crossed by three transverse ridges, at each end of which are the elliptical concave articular facets for the third to the sixth costal cartilages. Above is a demi-facet for the second and below a similar demi-facet for the seventh cartilage. The posterior aspect is smooth and slightly concave in its long axis.

The xiphoid is a slender, elongated process. It is usually only partially ossified.

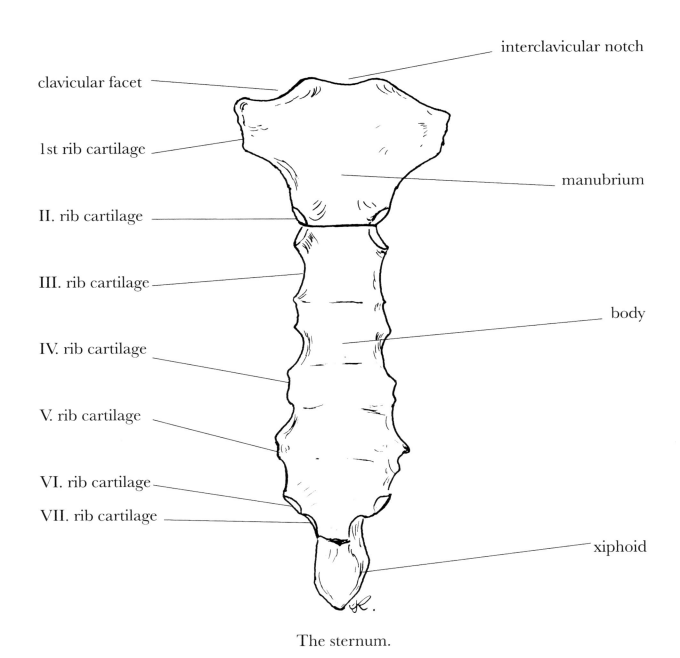

The sternum.

The sternum articulates with the clavicles, and seven costal cartilages on each side. It gives attachment to ten muscles – sternocleidomastoid, sternothyroid, sternohyoid, diaphragm, pectoralis major, transversus thoracis, transversus abdominus, aponeurosis of the external and internal obliques, and the rectus abdominus.

Practical fact – The sternum is a very strong bone and requires a great deal of force to fracture it. The principal danger lies not in the fracture itself, but the possibility that the broken bones may be pushed inwards, and damage the heart which lies immediately behind it.

THE RIBS

The twelve pairs of dorsal costal processes remain as separate arched bones, extending from the vertebral column in to the body wall and bounding the cavity of the thorax laterally. Each rib originates as a strip of cartilage, which for most part ossifies ectosteally, but its ventral extremity remains permanently as gristle so each rib consists of a bony and cartilaginous segment. The first to the seventh unite medioventrally with the sternum and are called true ribs and are classified as vertebro-sternal the eighth, ninth and tenth articulate with their respective predecessors and are known as vertebro-chondral, while the floating ribs, eleven and twelve are termed vertebral, as their ventral ends are free in the muscle of the body wall. The head of each rib shows a cartilage – covered facet on its extremity. In all but the 1st, 10th, 11th and 12th, this is divided into two by a transverse ridge (crista-capituli), the lower or primary facet being the larger, to articulate with the vertebra which corresponds to the rib in number: the upper or secondary facet being smaller to articulate with the vertebra above. The single facet on the above named ribs are in series with the lower facets on the others. Joining the head and body is a flattened neck, which present a sharp ridge directed upwards, crista colli superior, a smooth front, and a very rough back. Where the neck joins the body a tubercle projects backwards and downwards, bearing an articular surface, which rests on the transverse process of the vertebra corresponding to the rib in number. The two floating ribs have no tubercles, that of the 10th is rudimentary with no articular surface, that of the 9th has a very small irregular surface, and that of the 1st is directed backwards.

The body is a thin curved band of bone, with a concave, smooth surface directed inwards, and a convex rougher outer surface, a roundish edge directed upwards and a grooved border, with a sharp external edge directed downwards; the subcostal groove accommodating the intercostal vessels and nerve.

A short distance from the neck, its shaft is suddenly bent forwards making an angle, the hinder surface of which is rough for the attachment of the ilio-costalis tendon. The anterior end of the body is broader, thinner, porous and hallowed to receive the end of the costal cartilage.

The ribs are curved around two axis. Besides the main curve around the vertical axis, there is a secondary curve around a transverse axis; this increases from above downwards, causing an increased obliquity in the ribs.

When any rib except the first and second is laid with its lower edge on the table, its vertebral end rises, and its lower edge only touches the table at two places. Most of the ribs from the fourth to the tenth have a crista colli inferior as well as one above. On the fourth to the ninth, for a short distance above the tubercle there is a shallow sulcus costallis superior looking backwards, formed by the upward prolongation of the upper margin to which is attached the anterior transverse-costal ligament. The angle and tubercle are coincident in the first rib, but the distance between these points increases from above downwards. The ribs increase in length from the first to the eighth, then rapidly diminish to the twelfth.

First Rib

The first rib is very short, is the most curved, it is broad and flat, its surfaces facing upwards and outwards, and its borders inwards and outwards. It is placed obliquely in the body extending downwards and forwards from its vertebral to its sternal end. Its upper surface presents; 1st a rough area for the insertion of scalenus medius, 2nd and oblique groove for the lower trunk brachial plexus C8. T1 and the subclavian artery, 3rd a small rough area which ends at the inner border of the rib in a small projection, the scalene tubercle (**tubercle of Lisfranc**) for insertion of scalenus anterior 4th in front of this tubercle is an oblique groove for the subclavian vein, 5, anterior to the groove is a ridge for the costo-clavicular ligament and more anteriorly a roughness for the subclavius. The under surface is smooth and has no costal groove. The head is small and bears a single articular circular facet for the body of the first thoracic vertebra.

The neck is long, rounded and directed upwards, backwards, and laterally. At the tubercle the rib is bent, so that the head of the bone is directed slightly downwards; the angle and tubercle therefore coincide. The outer border of the rib is thin anteriorly but thicker posteriorly and is covered by the scalenus posterior as it descends to be inserted into the upper surface of the second rib. The inner border gives attachment to the supra pleural membrane, (**Sibson's fascia**) which covers the cervical dome of the pleura.

The remaining atypical ribs are the second, tenth, eleventh and twelfth.

Lisfranc de St Martin, J. (1790 – 1847).

Sibson, F. (1814 – 1876)

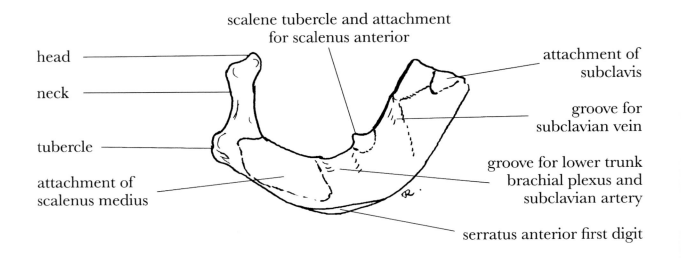

head

neck

tubercle

attachment of
scalenus medius

scalene tubercle and attachment
for scalenus anterior

attachment of
subclavis

groove for
subclavian vein

groove for lower trunk
brachial plexus and
subclavian artery

serratus anterior first digit

The first rib right side. Superior aspect.

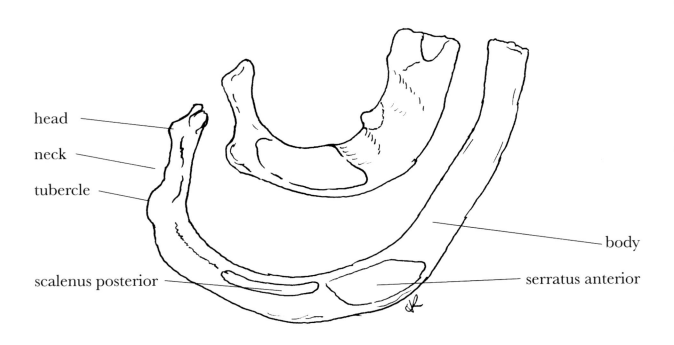

head

neck

tubercle

scalenus posterior

body

serratus anterior

The right, first and second ribs.

Robson's Approach To Anatomy

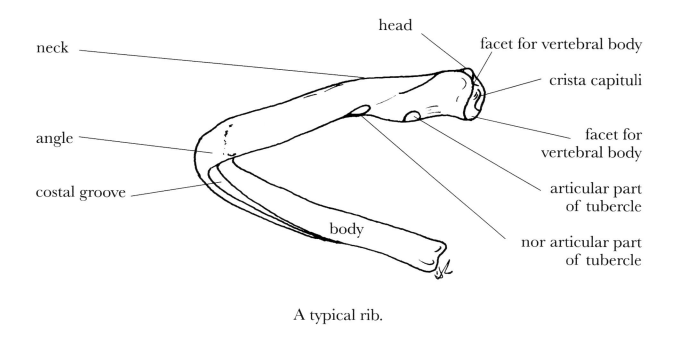

neck

head

facet for vertebral body

crista capituli

facet for
vertebral body

angle

articular part
of tubercle

costal groove

nor articular part
of tubercle

body

A typical rib.

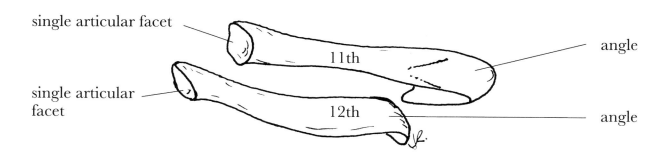

single articular facet

angle

11th

single articular
facet

angle

12th

The eleventh and twelfth ribs, posterior aspect.

The costal cartilages – The rib cartilages resemble in shape the sternal ends of the bony ribs, they are bars of hyaline cartilage, each is enveloped in a thick perichondriuim. That of the first is short, thick and irregular, and like that of the second and third is continued forward in the line of the rib, the fourth to seventh which is the largest is also connected to the sternum. The cartilages of the eighth, ninth and tenth ribs are connected to the inferior border of the cartilage immediately above. The eighth cartilage is occasionally, but rarely prolonged to the sternum, if so, it is more on the right than the left. The eleventh and twelfth are pointed and end in the posterior abdominal wall.

Practical fact:- in old age they are prone to ossify in endostosis.

THE THORAX

The skeleton of the thorax is an osseocartilaginous cage which contains and protects the principal organs of circulation and respiration. It is conical in shape, narrow above and broad below. Flattened from before backwards and longer posteriorly than anteriorly.

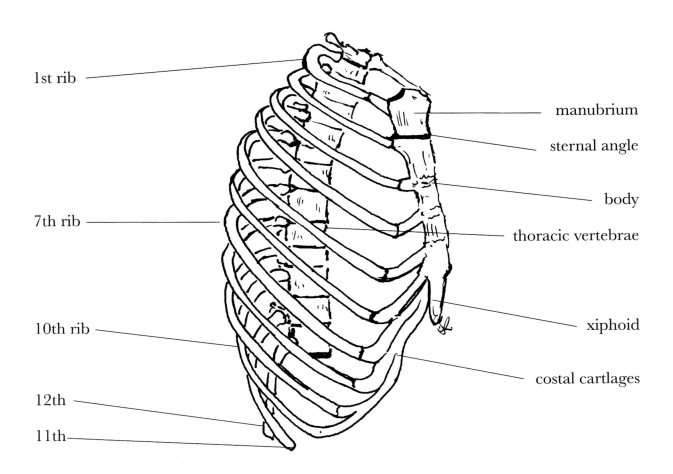

1st rib
7th rib
10th rib
12th
11th

manubrium
sternal angle
body
thoracic vertebrae
xiphoid
costal cartlages

Thoracic cage, right side.

Boundaries – Posteriorly it is formed by the twelve thoracic vertebrae and posterior parts of the ribs. Anteriorly the sternum and costal cartilages, laterally it is convex and is formed by the ribs, the ribs and costal cartilages are separated from each other by the intercostal muscles and membranes. The thoracic inlet slopes downwards and forwards, it is bounded posteriorly by the body of the first thoracic vertebra, anteriorly by the manubrium sterni and laterally by the first rib on each side. The thoracic outlet is bounded posteriorly by the twelfth thoracic vertebra, laterally by the eleventh and twelfth ribs, and anteriorly by the costal cartilages of the seventh, to tenth ribs. The thoracic outlet is wider transversely from before backwards and slopes obliquely downwards and backwards, it is closed by the diaphragm which forms the floor of the thorax, and separates the contents of the thoracic from the abdominal cavity.

THE APPENDICULAR SKELETON

The bones of the upper limb are divisible into four groups. i) The shoulder girdle – clavicle and scapula. ii) The upper arm – humerus.   iii) The forearm – radius and ulna.   iv) The hand – eight carpals forming the wrist, five metacarpals forming the palm, fourteen phalanges, three in each finger, two in the thumb and two sesamoid bones at the base of the proximal thumb phalanx.

The Clavicle

Stretches obliquely upwards, backwards and outwards from the manubrium sterni to the acromion process of the scapula.   It is curved like and italic f with its inner concavity directed backwards and its outer forwards, its lateral end bears a transversely elongated but rarely smooth facet to articulate with the acromion.   The outer third is flattened above and presents a rough concave anterior margin from which the deltoid arises, and a convex posterior edge which with part of the adjoining superior surface gives insertion to the trapezius, and projects into a prominent coracoid angle which overlies the coracoid process. The inferior surface of this angle there is a rough conoid tubercle, from which a short coarse trapezoid ridge runs outwards and forwards.   These give attachment to the coraco-clavicular ligaments.   For the inner two-thirds the clavicle is rounder and its back directed concavity arches over the subclavian vessels and the brachial plexus, its superior surface is covered by the platysma.   The medial two-thirds constitute the prismoid portion of the bone.   The anterior surface of the sternal half gives origin to the clavicular portion of the pectoralis major, the rough medial one-third posterior border superior surface gives origin to the clavicular head of sternocleidomastoid.   The sternal end is triangular in form and is directed medialwards, and a little downwards and forwards.   On its articular facet which is concave from before backwards, and convex from above downwards, it articulates with the articular disc of the sternoclavicular joint. From the lower and back part of the bone lateral to this articular surface the sternohyoid arises.

The inferior surface is rough and conspicuously ridged.   Internally where it overlies the costal cartilage of the first rib there is a costal tuberosity for the costoclavicular ligament, lateral to which the surface is grooved as far as the conoid tubercle for the insertion to the subclavius muscle; the clavipectoral fascia splits to enclose the muscle and is attached to the margins of the groove.

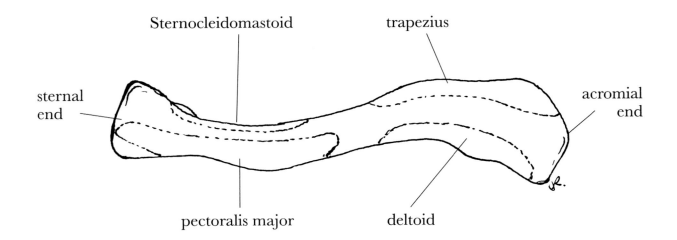

The left clavicle, superior surface.

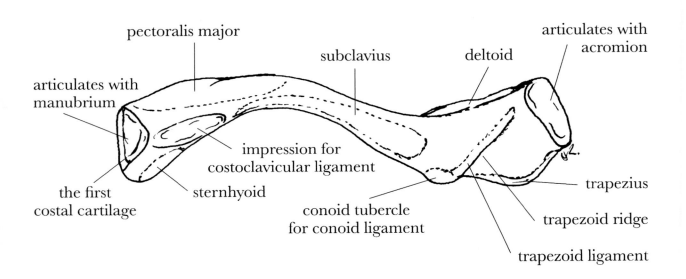

The left clavicle, inferior aspect.

The clavicle articulates with three bones, manubrium sterni, scapula, and first rib. It gives attachment to six muscles, sternocleidomastoid, deltoid, pectoralis major, subclavius, trapezius and sternohyoid.

The Scapula

The scapula is a flat trianglar bone placed on the posterior surface of the thorax between the second and seventh ribs, from which it is separated by the serratus anterior and areolar tissue. It has three borders, a short, sharp, concave upper, a long convex medial (vertebral), and a thick lateral (axillary); three angles – a thin sharp superior, a long rounded inferior, and a thick lateral or articular, and two surfaces – an anterior or costal presenting a concavity the subscapular fossae, and a posterior or dorsal divided by a strong ridge the spine, into two fossae the supraspinous and a infraspinous, these fossae communicate with each other through the spino-glenoid notch.

Borders – The superior border is sharp and thin, slopes upwards to the superior angle. It is marked at its lateral end by the suprascapular notch. The medial (vertebral) border is the longest of the three, and is divided into three areas; (1) from superior angle to the spine, for the levator scapulae, (2) a small triangular area at root of spine for the rhomboid minor, (3) from the lower part of the root to the inferior angle for the rhomboid major.

The lateral border is thickest dorsally it has a rough triangular area at the inferior angle for the teres major, from this to the lateral angle is an elongated impression for the teres minor, its upper part presents a groove for the circumflex scapular artery. Immediately below the glenoid is a rough tubercle the infra-glenoid, for the long head of triceps.

Angles – The superior is almost a right angle; the inferior is acute and often affords attachment slip of latissimus dorsi; the lateral angle constitutes the head of the bone. It is the largest and strongest, it is continuous with the body of the bone by a constricted part or neck. On the summit is a concave pear shaped facet the glenoid cavity, which is wider below than above, it articulates with the humerus. Above it is surmounted by the supra-glenoid tubercle for the long head of biceps.

Processes – The spine is a thick triangular process, projecting from the dorsal aspect of bone at junction of upper and middle third, its base forms a rounded concave border overlying the spino-glenoid notch, laterally the spine has a smooth area for the subtrapezial bursa. The acromion is the quadrilateral plate at the lateral part of the spine, its medial border bears an oval facet for the clavicle. The coracoid process, springs out from the top of the neck of the bone. The root of the process is short and vertical, the remainder or horizontal portion is directed forwards and slightly laterally. Its under surface is smooth and concave, the upper rough and convex.

Structures attached to coracoid process.

i)   Pectoralis minor – medial border of horizontal portion.

ii)   Coracobrachialis – medial part tip of horizontal portion.

iii)   Short head biceps – lateral part tip of horizontal portion.

iv)   Suprascapular ligament – medial border of root.

v)   Coracohumeral ligament – lateral border of root.

vi)   Coracoclavicular ligament – upper surface of horizontal portion.

vii)   Coracoacromial ligament – lateral border of horizontal portion.

viii)   Clavipectoral fascia – medial border of horizontal portion.

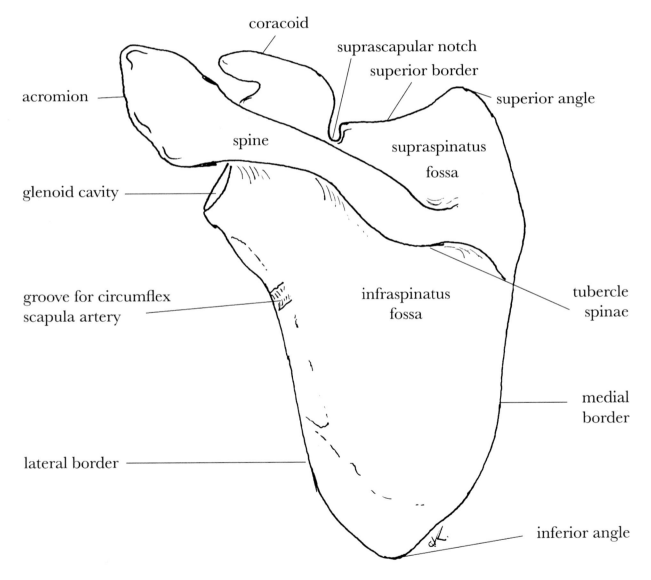

Left scapula, dorsal surface.

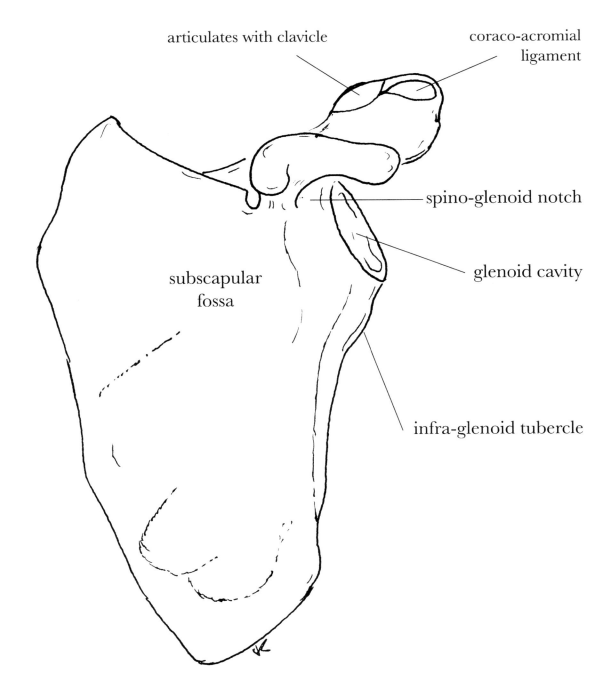

articulates with clavicle

coraco-acromial
ligament

spino-glenoid notch

subscapular
fossa

glenoid cavity

infra-glenoid tubercle

Left scapula, costal surface.

The scapula articulates with two bones, clavicle and humerus.   It gives attachment to seventeen muscles, costal surface – subscapularis, dorsal surface – infraspinatus, supraspinatus, spine – trapezius and deltoid, superior border – omo-hyoid inferior belly, medial border, serratus anterior, rhomboid minor et major, and levator scapulae from superior angle to triangular smooth area, lateral border – triceps, teres minor et major, corocoid process, short head of biceps, coracobrachialis, pectoralis minor, supraglenoid tubercle – long head of biceps.   Occasionally the latissimus dorsi has an attachment to the dorsi surface inferior angle.

The Humerus

Is the longest and largest bone of the upper extremity, articulating above with the scapula, below with the radius and ulna. It consists of a proximal end, a shaft and a distal end. The proximal end comprises a head, anatomical neck, surgical neck, two tuberosities and a bicipital groove. The shaft exhibits three borders, anterior, medial and lateral, together with three surfaces, namely antero-medial, antero-lateral, and posterior. The distal end is made up of two articular areas, the capitulum and trochlear; two eminences, the medial and lateral epicondyles, three fossae, radial, coronoid and olecranon .

The proximal end – The head is almost hemispherical in form articulating with the glenoid cavity of the scapula. Just below the periphery of the head is a faintly marked groove, the anatomical neck, which affords attachment of the capsule of the shoulder joint. The tuberosities greater and lesser are separated from each other by the upper part of the intertubercular sulcus. The shaft is cylindrical above and prismatic below. The posterior surface is convex from side to side, and impressed by the radial (musculo-spiral groove).

The distal end – This portion of bone curves forwards and is flattened from before backwards. The trochlear or medial articular area is pulley shaped and articular for the ulna. The capitulum, or lateral articular facet is for the head of the radius.

The medial epicondyle is a pyramid process. At the back is a shallow vertical groove for the ulnar nerve, from anterior aspect of this epicondyle is the common flexor origin.

The lateral epicondyle is a rough tubercle for several muscles, common extensor origin. Anteriorly are two hollows, one above the capitulum, the radial fossa, posteriorly is a much larger and deeper depression, the olecranon fossa.

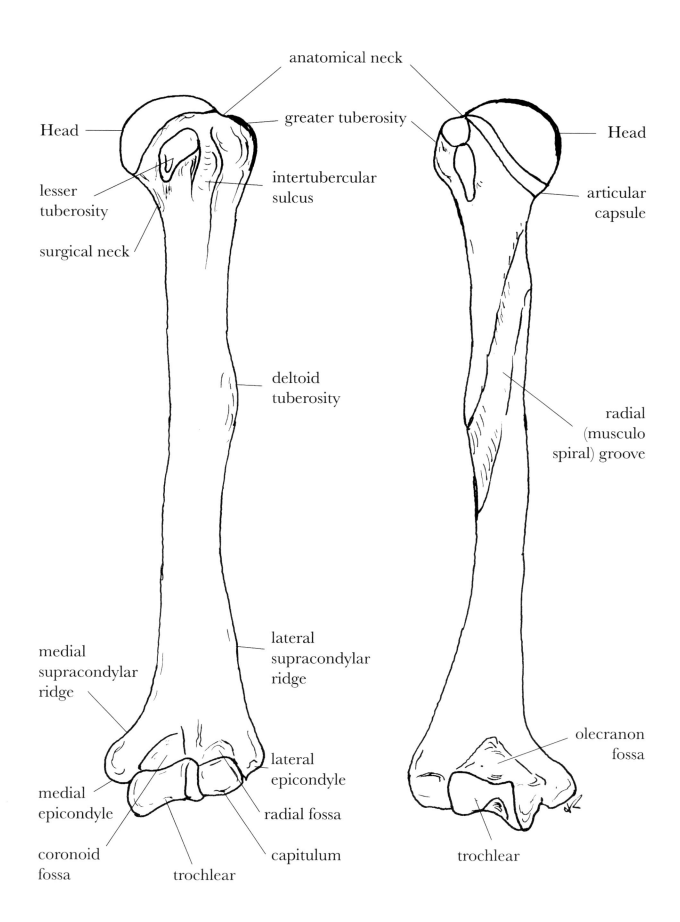

anatomical neck

Head

greater tuberosity

lesser
tuberosity

intertubercular
sulcus

surgical neck

Head

articular
capsule

deltoid
tuberosity

radial
(musculo
spiral) groove

medial
supracondylar
ridge

lateral
supracondylar
ridge

olecranon
fossa

medial
epicondyle

lateral
epicondyle

radial fossa

coronoid
fossa

capitulum

trochlear

trochlear

The left humerus

The Humerus

The humerus gives attachment to twenty four muscles, greater tuberosity, supraspinatus, infraspinatus, teres minor, lesser tuberosity, subscapularis.   Lateral lip of intertubercular sulcus, pectoralis major, medial lip of intertubercular sulcus, pectoralis major, medial lip of intertubercular sulcus, teres major.   Floor of the intertubercular sulcus – latissimus dorsi. Shaft, brachialis, coracobrachialis, deltoid, from posterior surface, medial and lateral heads triceps. medial epicondyle just above pronator teres.   Common flexor origin, medial epicondyle, flexor carpi radialis, palmaris longus.   Flexor digitorum superficialis. Flexor carpi ulnaris. Lateral supracondylar ridge, brachiordialis, extensor carpi radialis longus. Common extensor origin lateral epicondyle, extensor carpi radialis brevis, extensor digitorum communis, extensor digiti minimi, extensor ulnaris, posterior surface lateral epicondyle, anconeus, supinator.

The Radius

Is the lateral of the two bones of the forearm and consists of a proximal and distal end and a shaft. The proximal end comprises head, neck and a tuberosity. Three margins, medial, anterior and posterior, mark out the shaft into three surfaces, anterior, posterior and lateral, the distal end shows five surfaces, anterior, posterior, medial and lateral, also an ulna notch, a styloid process and a dorsal tubercle.

Proximal end – The head is the disc shaped process of the bone placed on top of the neck. Its upper surface is smooth, having a raised edge surrounding a central depression. The vertical circumference of the head is also smooth being deeper on the medial than the lateral side. The upper surface articulating with the capitulum of the humerus and the rim with the radial notch of the ulna being retained in this position by the annular ligament.

Shaft – The medial or interosseous border is the best marked.

Distal end – The posterior surface is grooved longitudinally for the several extensor tendons. About the middle is the dorsal radial tubercle (Lister) separating the groove for the tendon of extensor pollicis longus on the ulna side from that lodging the tendon of extensor carpi radialis brevis laterally.

Lister, J. (1827 – 1912).

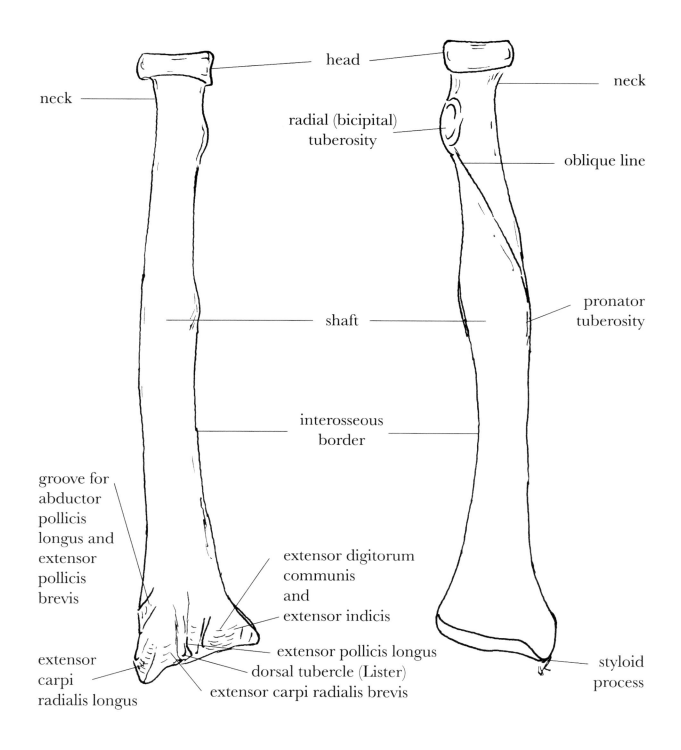

neck

head

neck

radial (bicipital)
tuberosity

oblique line

shaft

pronator
tuberosity

interosseous
border

groove for
abductor
pollicis
longus and
extensor
pollicis
brevis

extensor digitorum
communis
and
extensor indicis

extensor pollicis longus

extensor
carpi
radialis longus

dorsal tubercle (Lister)

extensor carpi radialis brevis

styloid
process

Posterior surface.   The radius.   Anterior surface.

The styloid process projects downwards from the lateral surface. The styloid process is rudimentary before the twelfth year. The ulna notch is medial and articular, semilunar in shape, concave from before backwards, and flat from above downwards, for the head of the ulna. The inferior surface is triangular in outline with the apex at the styloid process, is concave in all directions, smooth and articular. By a slight constriction it is divided into two areas; the lateral triangular for the scaphoid; and the medial quadrilateral for the lunate

The radius articulates with four bones, humerus, ulna, scaphoid and lunate and gives attachment to nine muscles. To radial tuberosity, biceps, anterior surface of shaft, flexor pollicis longus, pronator quadratus, oblique line, flexor digitorum superficialis and supinator. Lateral border, pronator tuberosity, pronator radii teres, styloid process brachioradialis, posterior surface of shaft, abductor pollicis longus, extensor pollicis brevis, supinator.

The Ulna

Is the medial of the two bones of the forearm, prismatic and larger above than below. It has proximal and distal ends and a shaft. The proximal end is made up of two notches, trochlear for articulation with the humerus and a radial notch for the head of the radius. The notches are bounded by the olecranon and coronoid processes. The shaft consists of an anterior, medial and posterior surfaces, separated by anterior posterior and lateral borders. The distal end consists of a head and a styloid process.

The ulna.

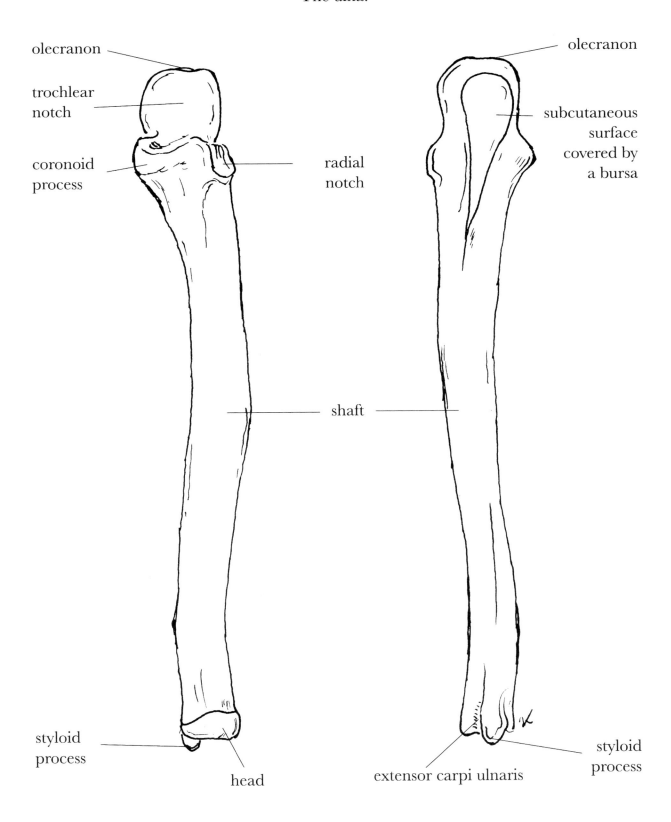

olecranon

trochlear notch

coronoid process

radial notch

shaft

styloid process

head

Anterior surface.

olecranon

subcutaneous surface covered by a bursa

shaft

extensor carpi ulnaris

styloid process

Posterior surface.

The ulna articulates with two bones. The humerus and radius and one articular disc. It gives attachment to fourteen muscles. To olecranonm triceps and anconeus. To coronoid process, flexor digitorum superficialis, pronator radii teres, brachialis and flexor pollicis longus, occasional head. Anterior surface of shaft, flexor digitorum profundus, pronator quadratus, posterior surface of shaft, anconeus, abductor pollicis longus. Extensor indicis, and aponeurosis, flexor carpi ulnaris and flexor digitorum profundus.

The Hand

The hand can be subdivided into three segments, the carpus or wrist, the metacarpals or palm, and the phalanges or fingers.

The carpals total eight in number and form two rows, a proximal and a distal.

From the radial to the ulna side the arrangement is:

Proximal row - Scaphoid, lunate, triquetral and pisiform.

Distal row - Trapezium, trapezoid, capitate and hamate.

The scaphoid articulates with five bones, radius, trapezium, trapezoid, capitate, lunate.

The lunate articulates with five bones, scaphoid, radius, capitate, hamate, triquetral.

The triquetral articulates with three bones, lunate, pisiform, hamate and the triangular inter-articular fibro-cartilage which separates it from the distal end of ulna.

The pisiform articulates with one bone, triquetral and gives attachment to two muscles, flexor carpi ulnaris, abductor digiti minimi.

The trapezium articulates with four bones, scaphoid, trapezoid, 1st and 2nd metacarpals , and gives attachment to three muscles, abductor pollicis brevis, oppenens pollicis, flexor pollicis brevis.

The trapezoid articulates with four bones, scaphoid, trapezium, cappitate, 2nd metacarpal, gives attachment to one muscle, part of flexor pollicis brevis.

The capitate articulates with seven bones, scaphoid, lunate, 2nd, 3rd and 4th metacarpals, trapezoid, hamate and gives attachment to one muscle, part of flexor pollicis brevis.

The hamate articulates with five bones, lunate, 4th and 5th metacarpals, triquetral, capitate and gives attachment to two muscles, flexor digiti minimi brevis, opponens digiti minimi.

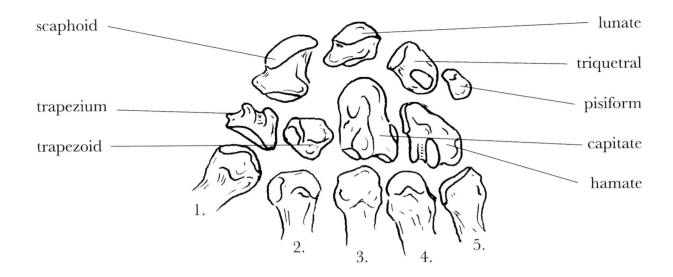

The right carpal bones and proximal metacarpals.

The metacarpal bones are five in number. The first is the shortest, the palmar surface of the head is impressed by two sesamoid bones.

The second is the longest.

The third has a styloid process projecting from postero-lateral angle of the base.

The fourth is the most slender

The fifth, presents a semilunar facet on its lateral side for the fourth metacarpal

The first metacarpal articulates with four bones, trapezium, proximal thumb phalanx and two sesamoid bones, and gives attachment to four muscles, opponens pollicis, abductor pollicis longus, radial head first dorsal interosseous, first palmar interosseous.

The second metacarpal articulates with five bones, trapezoid, trapezium, capitate, third metacarpal, and phalanx index finger. It gives attachment to six muscles, extensor carpi radialis, first dorsal interosseous ulna head. Second Palmar interosseous, radial head of second dorsal interosseous.

The third metacarpal articulates with four bones, capitate, second metacarpal, fourth metacarpal, proximal phalanx middle finger. It gives attachment to five muscles, Flexor carpi radialis, Extensor carpi radialis brevis, ulna head second dorsal interosseous, transverse and oblique heads of abductor pollicis.

The fourth metacarpal articulates with fives bones, hamates, capitate, third metacarpal, fifth metacarpal, proximal phalanx of ring finger. It gives attachment to three muscles, third palmar interosseous, ulna head third dorsal interosseous, radial head fourth dorsal interosseous.

The fifth metacarpal articulates with three bones, hamate, fourth metacarpal, proximal phalanx little finger. It gives attachment to four muscles, extensor carpi ulnaris, opponens digiti minimi, fourth palmar interosseous, ulna head of fourth dorsal interosseous.

The phalanges are fourteen in number, three for each finger and two for the thumb. Each proximal and middle phalanx articulates with two bones. The base of the proximal thumb phalanx gives attachment to six muscles, dorsal surface, extensor pollicis brevis. Lateral side, abductor pollicis brevis, flexor pollicis brevis, lateral part oblique head abductor pollicis, medial side transverse and remainder of oblique head adductor pollicis.

Base of proximal phalanx of little finger medial side, abductor digiti minimi, flexor digiti minimi, sides of each middle phalanx, flexor digitorum superficialis, base of dorsal surface, extensor digitorum communis, dorsal surface base of distal phalanges two to five, extensor digitorum communis, palmar surface flexor digitorum profoundus, dorsal surface distal phalanx thumb extensor pollicis longus, palmar surface flexor pollicis longus.

No muscle arises from any phalanx.

Robson's Approach To Anatomy

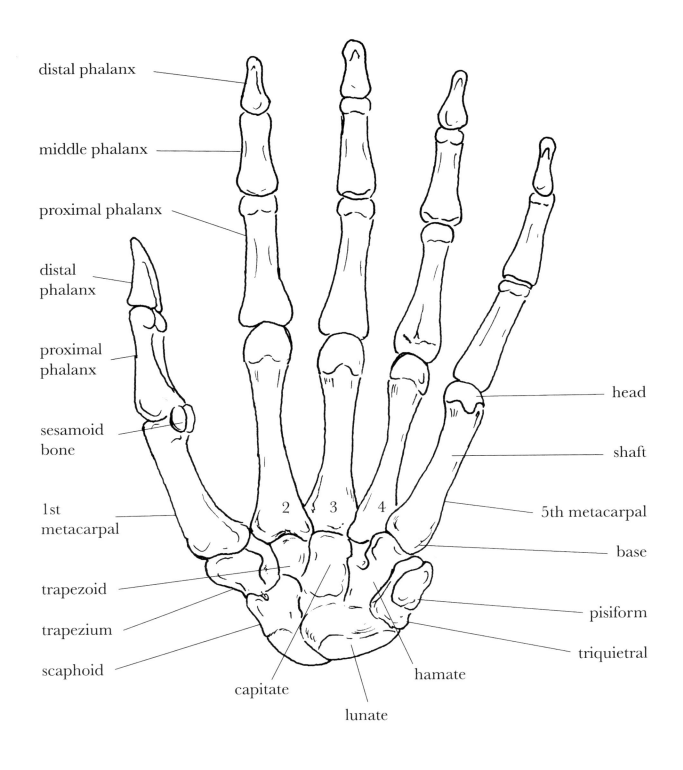

distal phalanx

middle phalanx

proximal phalanx

distal
phalanx

proximal
phalanx

sesamoid
bone

1st
metacarpal

trapezoid

trapezium

scaphoid

capitate

lunate

hamate

head

shaft

5th metacarpal

base

pisiform

triquietral

2   3   4

The left hand, palmar surface.

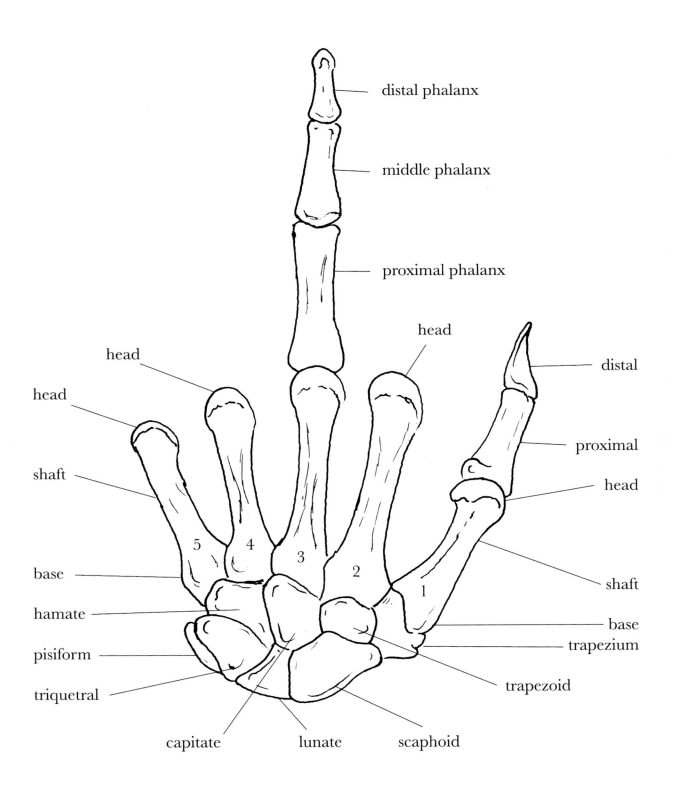

The carpals, metacarpals and phalanges, left hand, dorsal surface.

The hip bone, or os coxae, is large and irregularly shaped.   In part it belongs to the trunk and in part to the lower limb for it forms the pelvic girdle.   It consists in the child of three elements – a dorsal, the ilium which is the largest and articulates with the sacrum posteriorly; An anterior ventral, the pubis, which joins its fellow medially by synchondrosis; and a posterior ventral, the ischium.   There is a rudimental fourth or acetabular element, but it fuses with the others at an early age.   The ilium, ischium and pubis unite at the bottom of the large cup-shaped cavity the acetabulum and ankylose together in the adult.

The pubis and the ischium diverge from each other in front of the socket to re-unite again and thus form the boundaries of the obturator foramen.

The ilium articulates with its two fellow constituents of the hip bone, with the sacrum and femur; the other two elements articulate with the femur, the pubis also uniting with its fellow.   As a whole the hip bone articulates with three bones.   It gives attachment to thirty four muscles. Iliac crest, tensor fascia lata, external oblique, latissimus dorsi, internal oblique, transversus abdominus, quadratus lumborum, gluteus maximus. Anterior superior iliac spine – sartorius, anterior iliac spine – rectus femoris, straight head.   Posterior iliac spine, piriformis gluteal surface – gluteus maximus, gluteus medius, gluteus minimus, groove above acetabulum, rectus femoris reflected head.   Iliac fossa, - iliacus pubis, - pubic crest, - rectus abdominus, body, - adductor longus, gracilis, adductor brevis, inferior ramus, obturator externus.   Posterior surface, levator ani, obturator internus, superior ramus, - psoas minor, pectineus, inferior ramus, gracilis, adductor brevis, obturator externus, adductor magnus, obturator internus, sphincter urethrae.   Ischium – body – obturator externus, quadratus femoris.   Ischial tuberosity, long head of biceps, semitendinosus, semimembranosus, adductor magnus, inferior gemellus.   Ischial spine, - dorsal surface, - superior gemellus, pelvic surface, -levator ani, coccygeus.   Anterior surface ramus of ischium, - obturator externus, adductor magnus, gracilis.   Posterior surface pelvic aspect, - obturator internus, perineal surface, sphincter urethrae, part origin to ischiocavernosus, superficial transverse perneii.

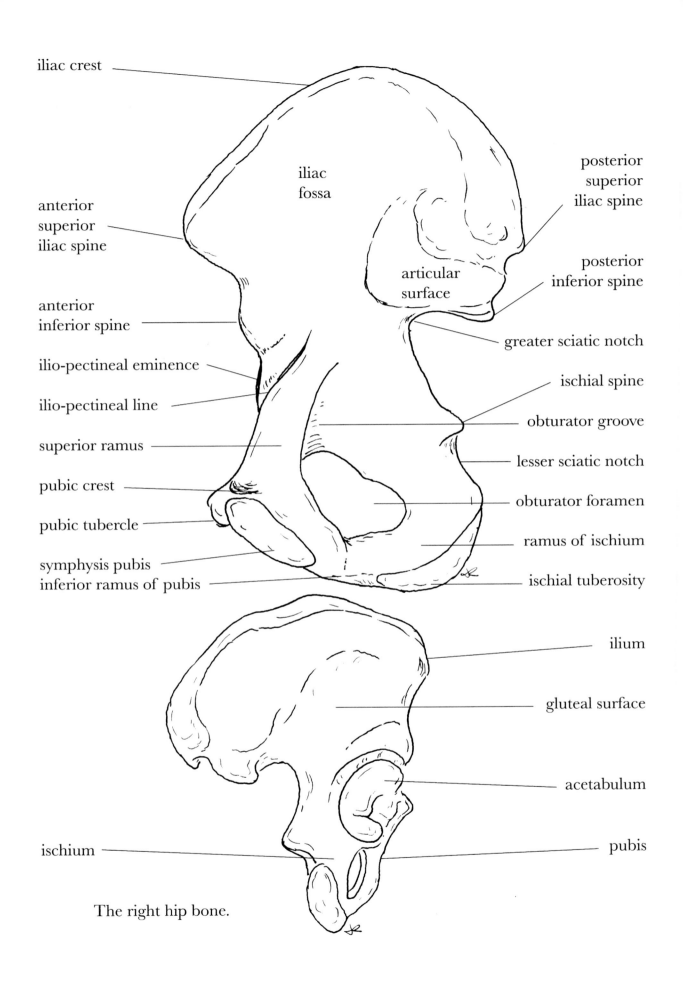

iliac crest

anterior
superior
iliac spine

anterior
inferior spine

ilio-pectineal eminence

ilio-pectineal line

superior ramus

pubic crest

pubic tubercle

symphysis pubis
inferior ramus of pubis

iliac
fossa

articular
surface

posterior
superior
iliac spine

posterior
inferior spine

greater sciatic notch

ischial spine

obturator groove

lesser sciatic notch

obturator foramen

ramus of ischium

ischial tuberosity

ilium

gluteal surface

acetabulum

ischium

pubis

The right hip bone.

Robson's Approach To Anatomy

THE PELVIS

The pelvis is composed of four bones; the two hip bones, sacrum and coccyx. The hip bones form the lateral and anterior boundaries; meeting each other in front to form the symphysis pubis; posteriorly they are separated by the sacrum. The interior of the pelvis is divided into a false and true pelvic cavity. The false pelvis is that part of the cavity which lies above the ilio-pectineal line and between the iliac fossae. This part belongs to the abdominal cavity and is in relation to the supra pubic and iliac regions.

The true pelvis is situated below the ilio-pectineal lines. The upper circumference, known as the superior aperature inlet or brim of the pelvis is bounded anteriorly by the tubercle and pectin of the pubis on each side, posteriorly by the anterior margin base of sacrum, and laterally the ilio-pectineal lines. The inlet in the normal pelvis is heart shaped being abtusely pointed in front, posteriorly it is encroached upon by the promontory of the sacrum. It has three principle diameters; **a**) Antero-posterior is measured from the sacro-vertebral angle to the symphysis-pubis. **b**) Transverse representing the greatest width of the pelvic cavity. **c**) Oblique is measured from the sacro-iliac joint of one side to the ilio-pectineal eminence of the other. The cavity of the true pelvis is bounded in front by the symphysis, behind by the sacrum and coccyx, laterally by a smooth wall of bone formed in part by the ilium and ischium. The cavity is shallow in front where it is formed by the pubes and deepest posteriorly.

The inferior aperture or outlet is very irregular and encroached upon by three bony processes, the posterior process is the coccyx, and two lateral processes, the ischial tuberosities. They separate three notches; **1**) The anterior notch is the sub-pubic arch, which is bounded on each side by the conjoined rami of the pubes and ischium. Each of the two remaining gaps are bounded by the ischium anteriorly, the sacrum and coccyx posteriorly, and the ilium above corresponds to the greater and lesser sciatic notches. These are converted into foramina by the sacrotuberous and sacro-spinous ligaments.

The axis of the pelvis – This is an imaginary line drawn at right angles to the planes of the brim, cavity and outlet through their central points.

Differences according to sex – There is a marked difference in size and form of the male and female pelvis. The various points of divergence may be tabulated as follows:-

	MALE	FEMALE
1	Bones stronger, heavier and have well marked muscular impressions	Bones more slender with slight muscular impressions
2	Ilia less vertical	Ilia more vertical
3	Iliac fossa deeper	Iliac fossa shallower
4	No preauricular sulcus	Preauricular sulcus
5	False pelvis relatively wider	False pelvis relatively narrower
6	True pelvis deeper True pelvis narrower	True pelvis shallower True pelvis wider
7	Inlet more heart shaped	Inlet more oval
8	Symphysis deeper	Symphysis shallower
9	Ischial tuberosities inverted	Ischial tuberosities everted
10	Pubic arch narrower and more pointed	Pubic arch more rounded
11	Margins of ischio-pubic rami more everted	Margins of ischio-pubic rami less everted
12	Obturator foramen oval	Obturator foramen triangular
13	Sacrum narrower and more curved	Sacrum wider and less curved
14	Capacity of true pelvis less	Capacity of true pelvis greater
15	Acetabula closer together	Acetabula wider apart.

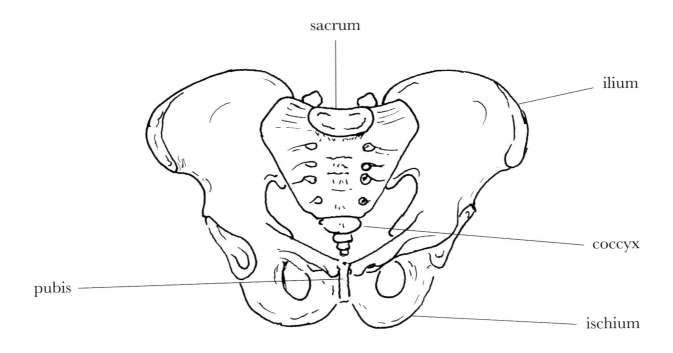

sacrum

ilium

coccyx

pubis

ischium

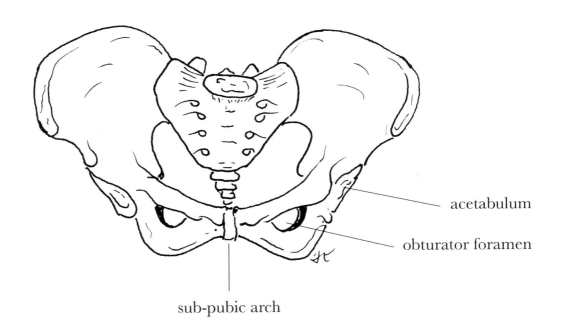

acetabulum

obturator foramen

sub-pubic arch

The male and female pelvis.

THE FEMUR

The femur is the longest and largest bone in the skeleton, and transmits the entire weight of the trunk from the hip to the tibia. It consists of an upper end comprising, head, neck, greater and lesser trochanters, a shaft, and a lower end comprising of two masses of bone, the condyles.

The head is more than half a sphere, is directed upwards, medially, and slightly forward to articulate with the acetabulum. With the exception of a small rough depression, the fovea capitis, for the ligamentum teres, a little below and behind the centre of the head, its surface is covered by hyaline cartilage. The neck of the femur which is about 5cm long, connects the head and the shaft with which it forms an angle of about 125°, its anterior surface is in the same place with the front aspect of the shaft, but is marked off from it by a ridge to which the capsule of the hip joint is attached. The ridge which commences at the greater trochanter in a small prominence, the superior cervical tubercle, extends obliquely downwards to the inferior cervical tubercle between the cervical tubercles is the intertrochanteric line and immediately below the lesser trochanter is the pectineal line. The superior and inferior cervical tubercles receive the bands of the ilio femoral ligament. Y-shaped ligament of Bigelow[1]; the strongest ligament in the body. The posterior surface of the neck is smooth and concave and its inner two-thirds is enclosed in the capsule of the hip joint. The trochanters are two prominences and are known as the greater and lesser. The greater is a thick quadrilateral process surmounting the junction of the neck with the shaft. The medial surface presents a roughened depressed area, the trochanteric fossa, which receives the tendon of obturator externus. The upper border lies one hand's breadth below the tubercle on the iliac crest, and on a level with the centre of the head of the femur. The anterior surface of the trochanter presents a roughened impression; Its lateral surface is divided into two areas by an oblique, flattened strip wider above than below, which runs downwards and forwards across it. The lateral surface is palpable in the living. The lesser trochanter is a conical eminence projecting medially and backwards from the shaft at its junction with the lower and posterior part of the neck. The inter trochanteric crest, it is a smooth rounded ridge, commences at the posterosuperior angle of the Greater trochanter and passes downwards and medially to terminate at the lesser trochanter. At its middle is an elevator termed the quadrate tubercle. The body or shaft of the femur is almost cylindrical but is slightly flattened in front and is strengthened behind by a projecting longitudinal ridge, the linea aspera which has distinct medial and lateral lips separated by a narrow interval when followed into the upper third of the shaft; the three parts diverge. The outer lip becomes continuous with the gluteal tuberosity and ends at the base of the greater trochanter. The ridge affords attachment to the gluteus maximus, and when very prominent is termed the third trochanter. The inner lip curves inwards below the lesser trochanter where it is known as the linea pectinea, and becomes continuous with the spiral line; the intervening portion bifurcates and is continued upward as two lines, one of which ends at the lesser trochanter, whilst the other joins the quadrate tubercle. The latter is known as the linea quadrate. Towards the lower third of the shaft the medial and lateral lips of the lines aspera again diverge, and are continued downwards towards the femoral condyles by the

[1] **Bigelow, H.J.** (1818 – 1890)

medial and lateral supra-condylar lines, enclosing between them a triangular surface of bone, the popliteal surface of the femur, which forms the upper part of the floor of the popliteal fossa. The lateral supra-condylar line is the more prominent and terminates below at the lateral epicondyle. The medial supra-condylar line is interrupted above, where the femoral vessels are in relation with the bone, is better marked below where it terminates in the adductor tubercle, a small projection at the summit of the medial epicondyle. The lower end is widely expanded in order to provide a good bearing surface for the transmission of the weight of the body to the top of the tibia. It consists of the cartilage-covered condyles, separated posteriorly by the intercondylar fossa. The lateral condyle is wider than the medial and more prominent anteriorly; the medial is narrower, more prominent laterally, and longer to compensate for the obliquity of the shaft. When the femur is in the natural position, the inferior surfaces of the condyles are on the same plane, and almost parallel, for articulation with the upper surfaces on the upper surface of the tibia. The two condyles are continuous in front, forming a smooth trochlear surface for articulation with the patella. The surface presents a median vertical groove, and two lateral convexities, the lateral of which is wider, more prominent, and prolonged farther upwards. The patella surface is faintly marked off from the tibial articular surfaces by two irregular grooves best seen while the lower end is still coated with cartilage. The lateral groove commences on the inner margin of the lateral condyle near the front of the intercondylar fossa, and extends obliquely forwards and outwards to the outer margin of the bone. The general direction of the medial groove is from front to back, turning inwards in front and extending backwards as a faint ridge which mark off from the rest of the medial condyle a narrow semilunar facet for articulation with the medial perpendicular facet of the patella in extreme flexion. The grooves receive the semilunar fibro-cartilages (menisci) in the extended position of the joint. The opposed surfaces of the two condyles form the lateral boundaries of the intercondylar fossa and give attachment to the cruciate ligaments. The anterior cruciate ligament is attached to the flattened impression medial surface of lateral condyle, the posterior cruciate is attached to a larger impression on the lateral surface medial condyle. The medial epicondyle gives attachment to the tibial collateral ligament. The lateral epicondyle gives attachment to the fibular collateral ligament of the knee joint, above and behind it is a deep groove which receives the tendon of popliteus when the knee is flexed, and its anterior end terminates in a pit from which the tendon takes origin.

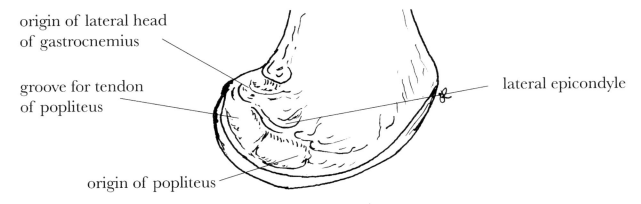

origin of lateral head
of gastrocnemius

groove for tendon
of popliteus

lateral epicondyle

origin of popliteus

The lateral aspect, distal end right femur.

The femur gives attachment to twenty three muscles – Greater trochanter, gluteus minimus et medius, piriformis, obturator internus, superior gemellus, inferior gemellus, obturator externus, quadratus femoris. Lesser trochanter, psoas major, iliacus. Shaft, posterior surface – vastus lateralis, gluteus maximus, biceps short head. Vastus medialis, adductor magnus, pectineus, adductor brevis, adductor longus. Shaft anterior surface – Vastus intermedius, articularis genu, medial and lateral condyles, gastrocnemius, lateral condyle posterior surface, plantaris, lateral aspect of lateral condyle, popliteus.

The Femur.

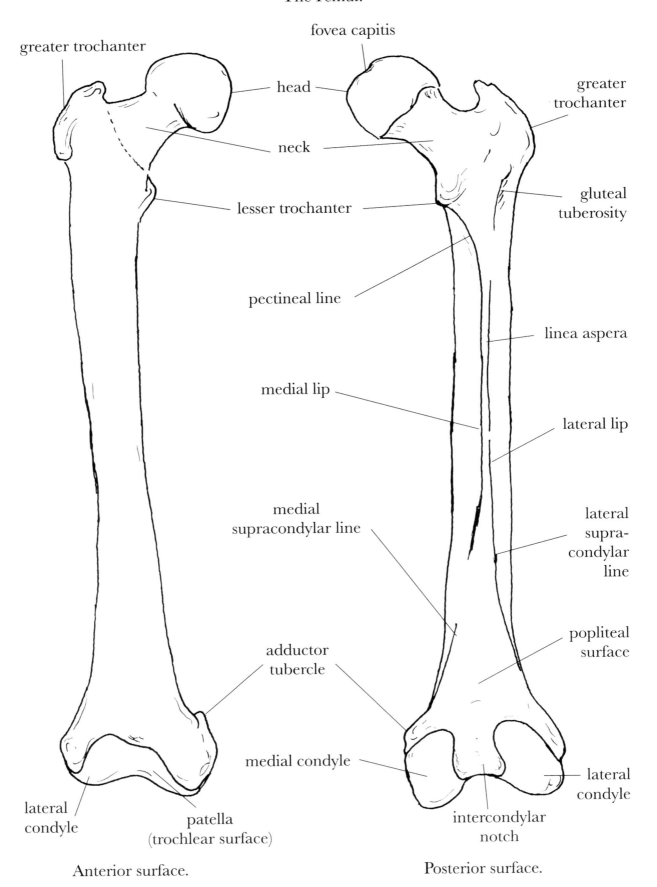

greater trochanter

fovea capitis

head

neck

lesser trochanter

pectineal line

medial lip

medial
supracondylar line

adductor
tubercle

medial condyle

lateral
condyle

patella
(trochlear surface)

Anterior surface.

greater
trochanter

gluteal
tuberosity

linea aspera

lateral lip

lateral
supra-
condylar
line

popliteal
surface

lateral
condyle

intercondylar
notch

Posterior surface.

THE PATELLA

The patella situated in from of the knee joint, is the largest of the sesamoid bones, is triangular in shape, and is developed in the tendon of the quadriceps femoris – Its anterior surface, marked by numerous longitudinal striae, is slightly convex, and perforated by small openings which transmit nutrient vessels to the interior of the bone. It is covered in the recent state by a few fibres prolonged from the common tendon of insertion (supra-patella tendon) of the quadriceps femoris into the ligamentum patellae (infra-patella tendon), and is separated from the skin by a bursa. The posterior surface is largely articular being smooth and divided into two facets by a vertical ridge, corresponding to the groove on the trochlear (patella) surface of the femur, into a large lateral facet for the lateral condyle of the femur, and a smaller facet for the medial condyle of the femur. Close to the inner edge a faint vertical ridge sometimes marks off a narrow articular facet, for the outer margin of the medial condyle in extreme flexion. Below the articular surface the apex which points downwards, is roughened in its lower part for the attachment of the ligamentum patellae. The superior border or base is thick, and sloped from behind backwards and forwards, and affords attachment, except near its posterior margin, to that portion of the quadriceps femoris, which is derived from the rectus femoris and vastus intermedius. The medial and lateral borders, are thinner than the base, converge to the apex below, and receive parts of the vasti medialis et lateralis. Near the junction of the base and lateral border there is a small shallow, circular depression into which part of the tendon of the vastus lateralis is inserted. The apex forms a blunt point directed downwards, and gives attachment to the ligamentum patellae which is attached to the upper portion of the tibial tuberosity. The patella is analogus to the olecranon process of the ulna.

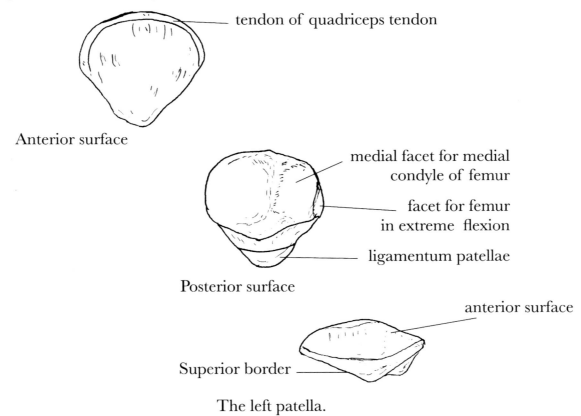

Anterior surface

tendon of quadriceps tendon

medial facet for medial condyle of femur

facet for femur in extreme flexion

ligamentum patellae

Posterior surface

anterior surface

Superior border

The left patella.

THE TIBIA

The tibia or shin bone, the name tibia has been used since ancient times when it referred to an assortment of musical instruments of long tubular form, made from the shin bones of animals and birds. It is situated at the front and medial side of the leg and nearly parallel with the fibula. Excepting the femur it is the largest bone in the skeleton, and alone transmits the weight of the trunk to the foot. It is prosmoid in form, and possesses a shaft and two ends. Its lower end is smaller than its upper end, and on its medial side a stout process, the medial malleolus, projects downwards beyond the rest of the bone. The tibia articulates above with the femur, below with the tarsus, and laterally with the fibula. The upper end is expanded especially in its transverse axis to provide a good bearing surface for the body weight transmitted through the lower end of the femur. It consists of two prominent eminences, named the medial and lateral condyles, superiorly each is covered with an articular surface, the two being separated by an irregularly roughened intercondylar area. The medial condyle is the larger, its upper articular surface, oval in outline, is concave in both diameters, and its lateral border projects upwards, deepening the concavity and covering an elevation named the medial intercondylar tubercle. The lateral condyle overhangs the shaft, especially at its posterolateral part, which bears on its lower surface a small circular facet for articulation with the upper end of the fibula. The upper surface is covered with an articular surface for the lateral condyle of the femur. It is circular in outline, slightly hollowed in its central part and its medial border extends upwards to cover an elevation named the lateral intercondylar tubercle. The anterior, posterior and lateral surfaces of the condyle are rough. The peripheral portion of each articular surface is overlaid by a fibro-cartilaginous meniscus of semilunar shape, connected with the margins of the condyles by bands of fibrous tissue termed coronary ligaments. Each meniscus is attached firmly to the rough interval separating the articular surfaces. This interval is broad and depressed in front, where it affords attachment to the anterior horns of the medial and lateral menisci and the anterior cruciate ligament; elevated in the middle to form the intercondyloid eminence or spine of the tibia, a prominent eminence presenting at its summit two compressed tubercles on to which the condylar articular surfaces are prolonged; the posterior aspect of the base of the eminence affords attachment to the posterior horns of the lateral and medial menisci, and limits a deep notch inclined towards the medial condyle, known as the posterior intercondyloid or popliteal notch. It separates the condyles on the posterior aspect of the head and gives attachment to the posterior cruciate ligament, and posterior ligament of the knee joint. Anteriorly, the two condyles are confluent, and form a somewhat flattened surface of triangular outline, the apex of which forms the tibial tuberosity. The tuberosity forms a low eminence, divided into an upper, smooth portion which gives attachment to the ligament patellae. The lower part can be felt through the skin from which is separated from the skin by the subcutaneous infrapatella bursa. The shaft of the tibia is thick and prismatic above, becomes thinner as it descends for about two-thirds of its length, and then gradually expands towards its lower end. It presents an anterior border, commences at the tuberosity of the tibia and runs downwards to the anterior margin of the medial malleolus. The medial border extends from the anterior end of the groove on the medial condyle and runs downwards to the posterior margin of the medial malleolus. The lateral or interosseous border. It commences in front of the fibular facet on the lateral condyle, and towards its termination bifurcates to enclose a triangular area for the attachment of the interosseous membrane uniting the lower ends of the tibia and fibula. The medial surface is bounded by the anterior border in front and behind by the medial border. The lateral surface is placed between the anterior and interosseous borders. The posterior surface is bounded by the interosseous and the medial borders. The lower end of the tibia is quadrilateral in shape and presents a strong process called the medial malleolus, projecting downwards, from its inner side. It possesses anterior, medial, lateral, posterior and inferior surfaces, the tibia is a very vascular bone. The tibia gives attachment to eleven muscles – Posterior surface medial condyle – semimembranosus. Lateral condyle – tibialis anterior, extensor digitrum longus (communis). Shaft medial surface, semitendinosus, gracilis, sartorius. Lateral surface – tibialis anterior, posterior surface, popliteus, soleus, flexor digitorum longus, tibialis posterior.

THE FIBULA

The Fibula is situated on the lateral side of the leg and in proportion to its length is the most slender of all long bones. It is placed nearly parallel to the tibia with which it is connected above and below. In man it is a rudimentary bone and bears none of the weight of the trunk, but is retained on account of the muscles to which it gives origin, and its participation in the formation of the ankle joint. Like other long bones it consists of a shaft and upper and lower ends. The upper end is of an irregular quadrate form, and has a flattened articular surface directed upwards, forwards and medialwards, for articulation with the lateral tibial condyle, which is inclined to the horizontal at an angle of about 40°. On the lateral side is a thick, rough prominence continued behind into a pointed eminence the styloid process, which projects upwards from the posterior part of the head, and gives attachment to the fibula collateral ligament of the knee and to the tendon of biceps femoris. The ligament divides the tendon into two parts, the remaining part of the head is rough for the attachment of ligaments and muscles. In front the anterior tubercle gives origin to the anterior ligament of the superior tibio-fibula joint. Just below the tubercle the highest fibres of peroneus longus arises, behind the styloid process is the posterior tubercle which gives origin to the posterior ligament of the superior tibio-fibula joint and a few fibres of the soleus muscle. The shaft of the fibula appears twisted at its lower fourth, it presents four borders, anterolateral, anteromedial, posterior lateral and posterior medial. It has a lateral surface, bounded by the anterior and posterior borders. Medial (anterior) surface, bounded by anterior and interosseous borders. A posterior surface which is the largest of the three, is placed between the interosseous and posterior borders. The lower end or lateral malleolus is pyramid in shape, it descends to a lower level than the medial malleolus and lies on a more posterior plane. It consists of four surfaces, its lateral surface is subcutaneous, the anterior is rough and continuous below with the inferior border, the posterior is marked by a broad groove with a prominent lateral border, and a medial surface which has a triangular articular facet for articulation with the lateral facet of the tibia. The fibula is essentially a bone of origin, giving rise to nine muscles and receiving the insertion of only one. Head of fibula, biceps femoris, soleus, peroneus longus.

Shaft; anterior surface, extensor digitorum longus, peroneus tertius, extensor hallucis longus, medial surface; soleus, tibialis posterior, flexor hallucis longus.   Lateral surface; peroneus longus, peroneus brevis.

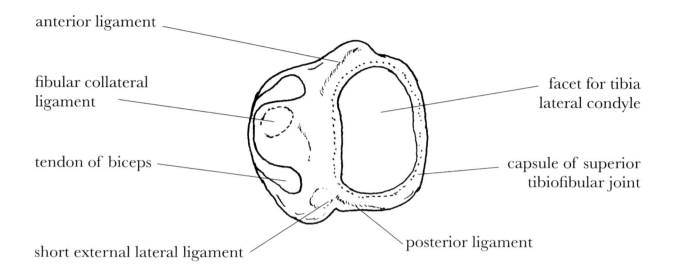

anterior ligament

fibular collateral ligament

tendon of biceps

short external lateral ligament

facet for tibia lateral condyle

capsule of superior tibiofibular joint

posterior ligament

The upper end of left fibula.

The tibia and fibula.

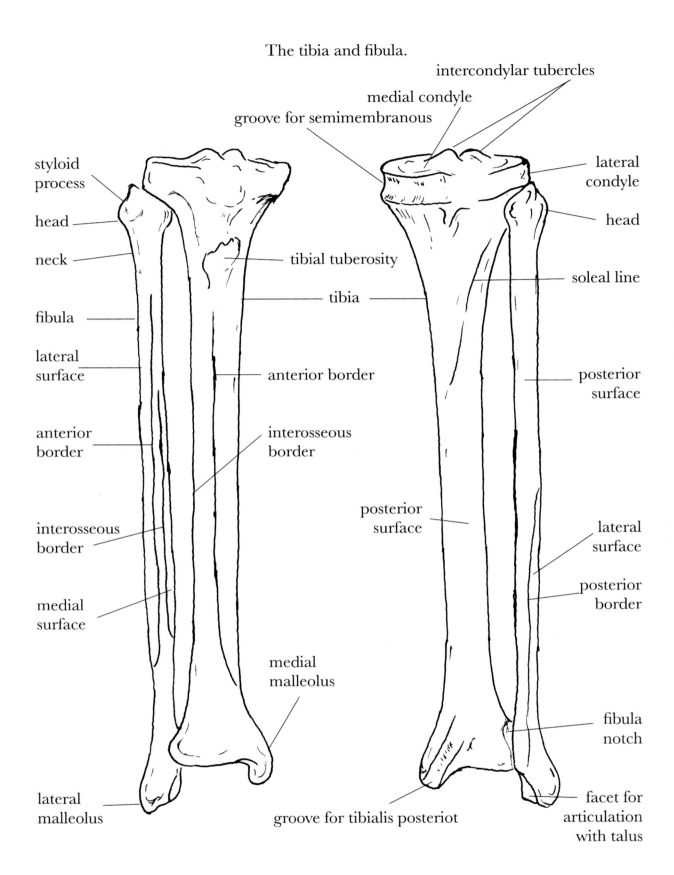

intercondylar tubercles

medial condyle

groove for semimembranous

styloid process

head

neck

fibula

lateral surface

anterior border

interosseous border

medial surface

lateral malleolus

tibial tuberosity

tibia

anterior border

interosseous border

medial malleolus

groove for tibialis posteriot

lateral condyle

head

soleal line

posterior surface

posterior surface

lateral surface

posterior border

fibula notch

facet for articulation with talus

Anterior surface.

Posterior surface.

THE FOOT

The bones of the foot in general arrangement correspond to the hand, differing in being modified for firmness not mobility.   The tarsal bones are grouped in three rows, a basal, consisting of the talus, and calcaneum, a central, the navicular, and a distal row consisting of the medial, intermediate and lateral cuneiforms, and the cuboid.   The metatarsals are five in number and form a closely united row, the phalanges are fourteen in number. **The talus** articulates with four bones – tibia, fibula, calcaneum and navicular, and gives attachment to no muscles.

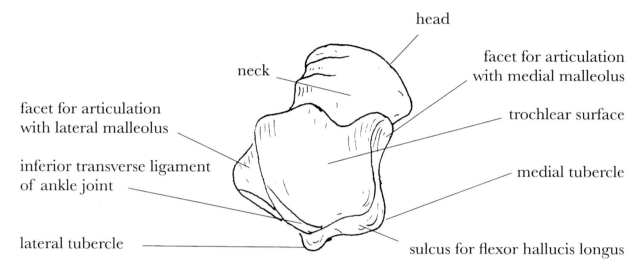

The talus, superior aspect.

The calcaneum – articulates with two bones, talus and cuboid, and gives attachment to eight muscles.   Gastrocnemius, soleus, plantaris via tendo-achilles.   Abductor hallicis, abductor digiti minimi, flexor digiti brevis, flexor accessorius, extensor digitorum brevis.

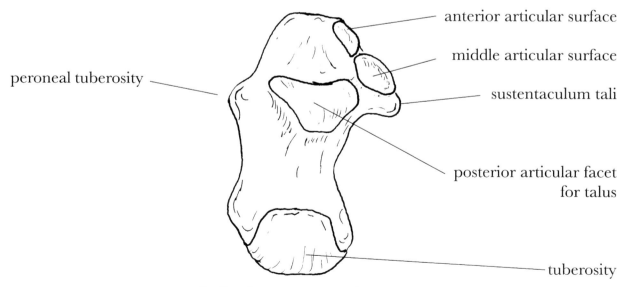

Left calcaneum, superior aspect.

The navicular - articulates with four bones, talus, medial, intermediate and lateral cuneiforms, occasionally with the cuboid on lateral side. It gives insertion to one muscle, tibialis posterior.

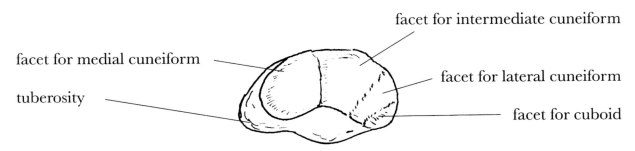

facet for intermediate cuneiform

facet for medial cuneiform

facet for lateral cuneiform

tuberosity

facet for cuboid

Left navicular, anterior view showing a facet for the cuboid.

The medial cuneiform - articulates with four bones, navicular, second cuneiform, second metatarsal and first metatarsal. It gives attachment to three muscles – tibialis anterior, tibialis posterior, peroneus longus.

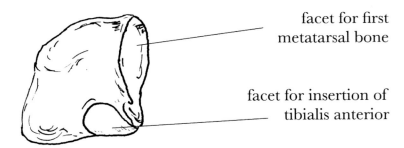

facet for first metatarsal bone

facet for insertion of tibialis anterior

Left medial cuneiform, lateral surface.

The intermediate cuneiform – articulates with four bones, navicular, second metatarsal, lateral cuneiform, and medial cuneiform. It gives attachment to one muscle – tibialis posterior.

The lateral cuneiform – articulates with six bones, navicular, third metatarsal, cuboid, fourth metatarsal, intermediate cuneiform, and second metatarsal. It gives attachment to two muscles – tibialis posterior, flexor hallucis brevis.

The metatarsals – the first metatarsal bone articulates with four bones, medial cuneiform, proximal phalanx, two sesamoid bones, It gives attachment to three muscles, tibialis anterior, peroneus longus, first dorsal interosseous.

The second metatarsal – articulates with five bones, medial, intermediate, lateral cuneiforms, third metatarsal, proximal phalanx. It gives attachment to three muscles, adductor hallucis, first and second dorsal interosseous.

The third metatarsal – articulates with four bones, lateral cuneiform, second and fourth metatarsals and proximal phalanx. It gives attachment to four muscles, adductor hallucis, second and third dorsal interosseous, first plantar interosseous.

The fourth metatarsal – articulates with four bones, cuboid, lateral cuneiform, fifth metatarsal, third metatarsal and proximal phalanx. It gives attachment to four muscles, adductor hallucis, third and fourth dorsal interosseous and second plantar interosseous.

The fifth metatarsal – articulates with three bones, cuboid, fourth metatarsal and proximal phalanx. It gives attachment to five muscles, peroneus brevis, peroneus tertius, flexor digiti minimi brevis, fourth dorsal interosseous and third plantar interosseous.

The phalanges – are fourteen in number, three in toes two to five and two in the first toe.

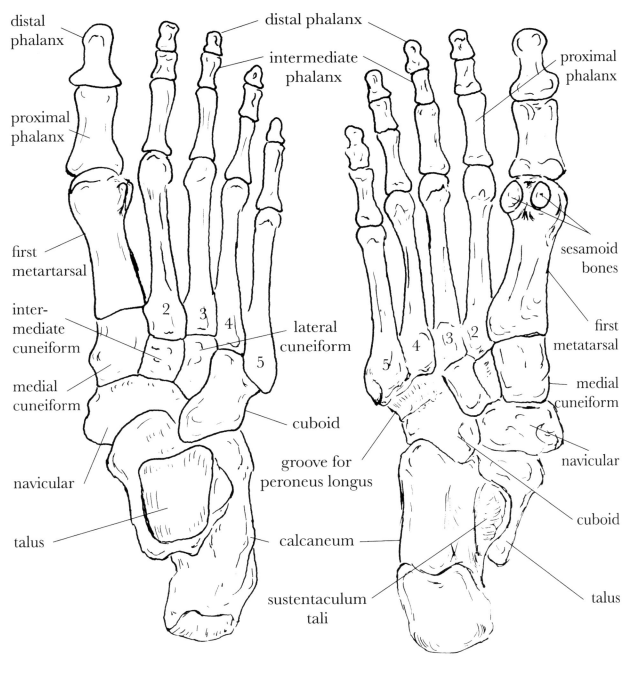

Dorsal surface.　　　　Plantar surface.
The right foot.

THE SKULL

The skull is the expanded upper portion of the axial skeleton and is supported on the summit of the vertebral column. It consists of the cranium, a strong, bony case enclosing the brain and is made up of eight bones – viz., occipital, two parietal, frontal, temporal, sphenoid and the ethmoid; and the bones of the face, surrounding the mouth and nose and forming with the cranium the orbital cavity for the reception of the eye. The bones of the face are fourteen in number – viz., two maxillae, two zygomatic (malar), two nasal, two lacrimal, two palatine, two inferior conchae (turbinates), the vomer and the mandible. All the bones enumerated above, with the exception of the mandible, are united by suture and are therefore immovable. A group of moveable bones comprising the hyoid suspended from the tips of the styloid process of the temporal bones, and three small bones, the incus, malleus, and stapes, situated in the middle ear or tympanic cavity, are also included in the enumeration of the bones of the skull. The skull is the bony skeleton of the head; it encases the brain, houses organs of special sense – viz., sight, smell, taste, hearing and touch. It helps form the first part of the respiratory and digestive tracts, many of the bones are hollow, reducing the weight of the skull and adding to the resonance of speech.

THE SKULL AT BIRTH

The most striking features of the skull at birth are its relatively large size in comparison with the body, and the predominance of the cranial over the facial portion of the skull. The frontal and parietal eminences are large and conspicuous; the sutures are absent; the adjacent margins of the bones of the vault are separated by septa of fibrous tissue continuous with the dura mater internally and the pericranium externally, hence it is difficult to separate the bones of the roof from the underlying dura mater, each side being lodged as it were in a dense membranous sac. The bones of the vault consist of a single layer without any diploe, and the cranial surfaces present no digital impressions. Six membranous spaces exist named fontanelles; two median called anterior and posterior, and two are present on each side called anterior and posterior lateral fontanelles. Each angle of the parietal bones is in relation with a fontanelle. The anterior fontanelle is lozenge-shaped, the posterior is triangular, the lateral are irregular in outline. Turning to the base, the most striking points are absence of the mastoid processes, and the large angle which the pterygoid plates form with the skull-base, whereas in the adult it is almost at a right angle. The base is relatively short and the lower border of the mental symphysis is on a level with the occipital condyles. The facial skeleton is relatively small in consequence of the small size of the nasal fossae, the small size of the maxillary sinus, and the rudimentary condition of the alveolar borders of the maxilla and mandible. The nasal fossae are as wide as they are high, and are almost filled with conchae. Growth takes place rapidly in the first seven years after birth, there is a second period of rapid growth at puberty when the air sinuses develop and this affects especially the face and frontal portion of the cranium.

Robson's Approach To Anatomy

The cranium at birth.

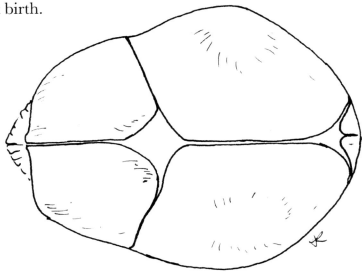

Superior aspect, showing anterior, and posterior fontanelles.

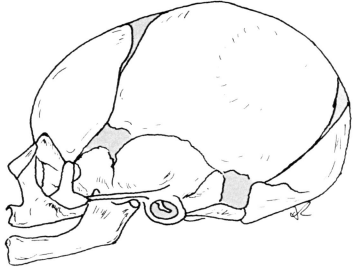

Lateral aspect, showing antero-lateral, and postero-lateral fontanelles

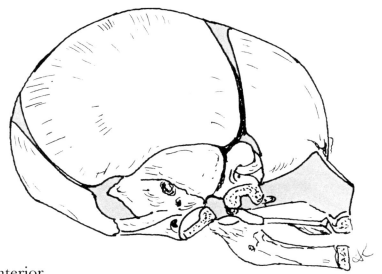

Sagittal section, interior

EPIPTERIC BONES

The epipterics are scale-like bones which occupy the antero-lateral fontanelles. Each epipteric bone is wedged between the squamo-zygomatic portion of the temporal, fontal, greater wing of sphenoid, and parietal, and it presents in most skulls between the second and fifteenth year. After that date it may present as a separate ossicle, or unit with the sphenoid, the frontal or squamo-zygomatic. The epipteric bone developed in membrane, and appears as a series of bony granules in the course of the first year.

WORMIAN BONES

Detached ossicles, known as wormian bones, are often to be seen in the lamboidal suture, and more rarely in any other sutures. These result from the presence of supernumeracy ossific centres, and are not to be confounded with the separate bones caused by want of union of normal centres. The persistence of the separation of the upper part of the supra-occipital and the lower part of the zygomatic are examples of the latter condition, and are not wormian bones.

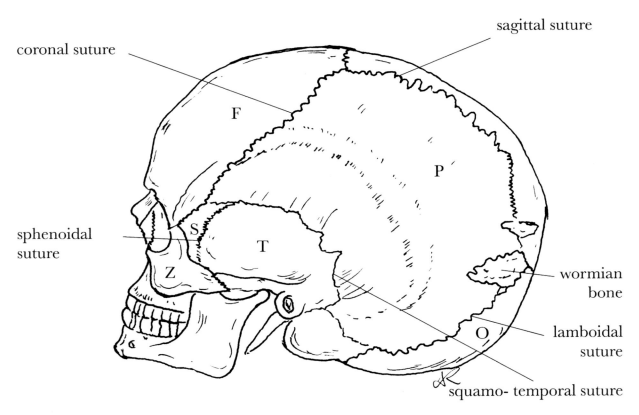

F - frontal bone
O - occipital bone
P - parietal bone

S - great wing of sphenoid bone
T - Temporal bone
Z - Zygomatic bone

The sutures of the cranium, showing the position of a wormian bone.

[1] **Worm, O.** (Olaus) (1588 – 1654).

THE FRONTAL BONE

The frontal bone is single, and forms the front of the cranium and is situated above the facial skeleton. It consists of four parts; squama frontalis, two orbital processes and a nasal spine. The frontal squama is the largest portion and forms the convexity of the forehead. The orbital plates project backwards, one from each supra-orbital margin, to form the roof of the orbit, and part of the floor or the anterior cranial fossae. The nasal spine projects downwards and forwards, extended on each side into two irregular alae, which articulate in front with the nasal bones, and on each side with the nasal processes of the maxillae and the lacrimal bone, posteriorly the ethmoid articulates. The frontal bone articulates with twelve bones, - viz., parietal, lacrimal, zygomatic, maxillae, nasal, ethmoid and sphenoid. Also the epipteric bones when present, occasionally with the squamous portion of the temporal. It gives origin to three pairs of muscles, - corrugator supercilli, orbicularis occuli, and temporalis. The frontal bone is ossified in membrane, from two primary centres which appear in the eighth week of intrauterine life, one for each half union begins in the second year.

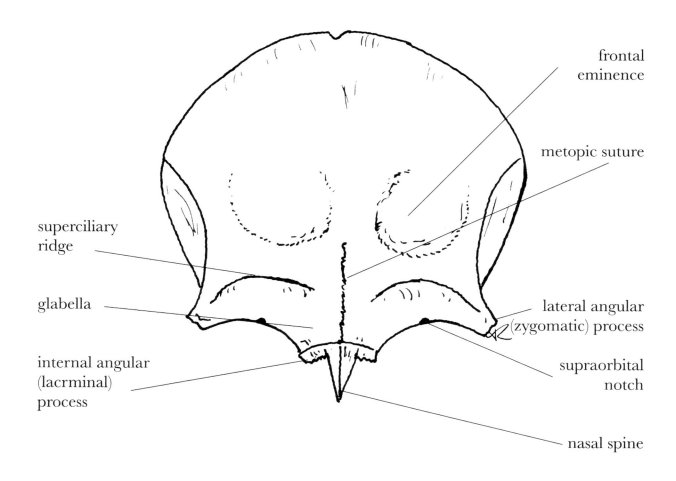

Frontal Bone, anterior surface.

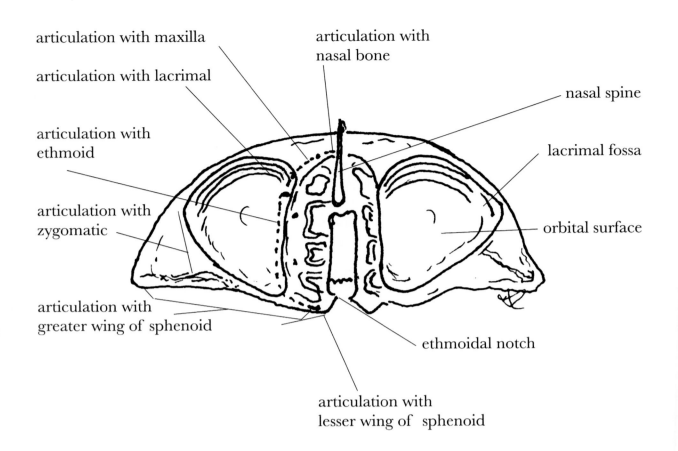

articulation with maxilla

articulation with lacrimal

articulation with
ethmoid

articulation with
zygomatic

articulation with
greater wing of sphenoid

articulation with
nasal bone

nasal spine

lacrimal fossa

orbital surface

ethmoidal notch

articulation with
lesser wing of sphenoid

Frontal bone, inferior surface.

THE PARIETAL BONES

The Parietal bones are two in number, symmetrical, and are interposed between the frontal bone before and the occipital bone behind. They form more than two-thirds of the roof and side walls of the cranium, they are quadrilateral in form, convex externally, concave internally and each has two surfaces, four borders and four angles. The parietal bone articulates with four bones., viz – frontal, sphenoid, temporal occipital, and its fellow of the opposite side. It gives origin to one muscle, temporalis.

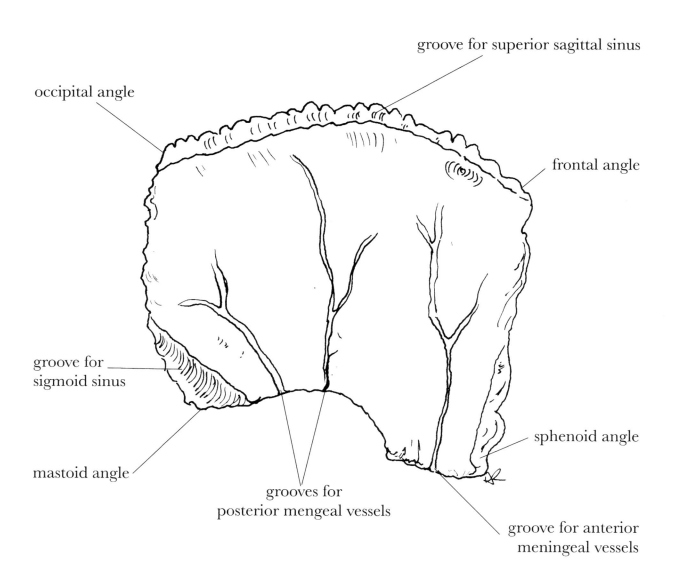

Left parietal bone, internal surface.

The parietal bone is ossified in membrane, from two centres, at the parietal eminence about the seventh week of intrauterine life.

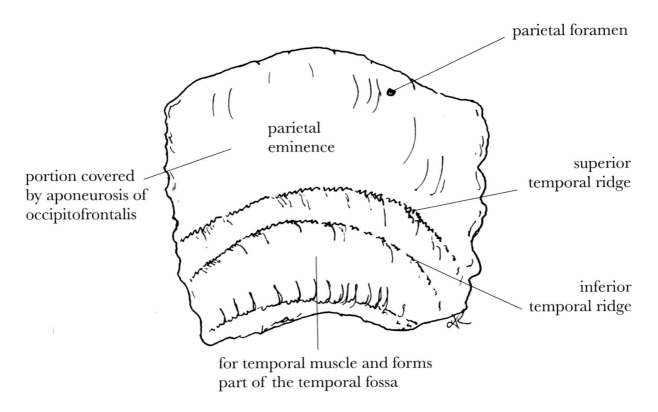

Left parietal bone, external surface.

THE OCCIPITAL BONE

The occipital bone is situated at the posterior and inferior part of the cranium. In general form it is flattened and trapezoid in shape, curved upon itself so that one surface is convex and directed backwards and somewhat downwards, while the other is concave and looks in the opposite direction. It is pierced in its lower and front part by a large aperture, the foramen magnum, by which the neural canal communicates with the posterior cranial fossa. It consists of four parts; basilar, squamous (tabular), and two condylar, so arranged the foramen magnum that the basilar part lies in front; The condylar parts on either side, and the squamous part above and behind. The occipital bone articulates by suture with two parietals, two temporals and the sphenoid bone; the condyles articulate with the atlas, and exceptionally the occipital articulates with the odontoid process of the axis. It gives attachment to thirteen muscles, highest nuchal line, occipital belly of Occipito-frontalis, superior nuchal line, Sternocleidomastoid, and Trapezius, space between superior and inferior nuchal lines, Semispinalis capitis, Spinalis capitis, Splenius capitis. Obliques superior capitis. Inferior nuchal line and

Space between it and foramen magnum, Rectus capitis posterior major, Rectus capitis posterior minor, basilar part, Longus capitis, Rectus capitis anterior, and Superior constrictor. Jugular process, Rectus capitis lateralis.

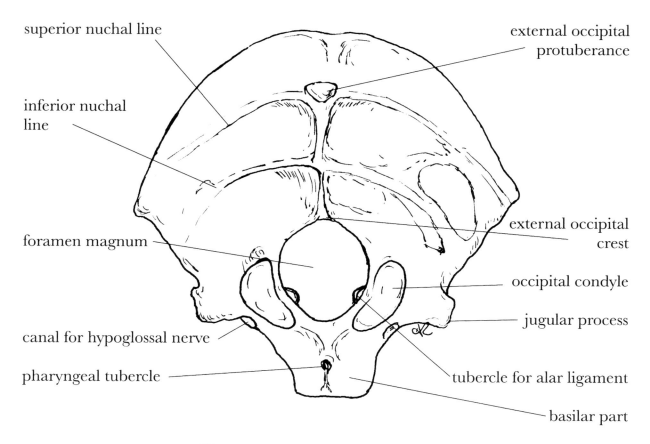

superior nuchal line

inferior nuchal line

foramen magnum

canal for hypoglossal nerve

pharyngeal tubercle

external occipital protuberance

external occipital crest

occipital condyle

jugular process

tubercle for alar ligament

basilar part

The occipital bone, external surface.

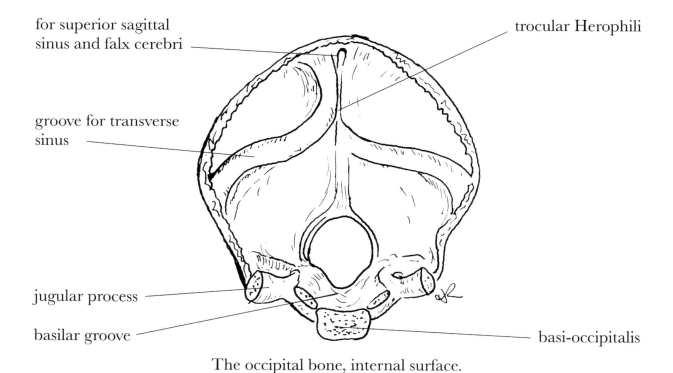

for superior sagittal sinus and falx cerebri

groove for transverse sinus

jugular process

basilar groove

trocular Herophili

basi-occipitalis

The occipital bone, internal surface.

Herophilus of Chalcedon, (c. 330 – 260 B.C.)

The occipital bone, at birth.

Interparietal portion
developed in membrane

The interparietal and
supra-occipital portions
form the squamous
portion in the adult

Supra-occipital
developed in cartilage

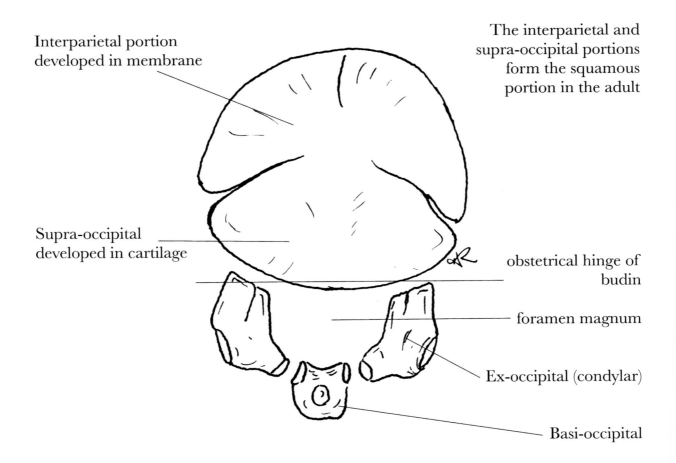

obstetrical hinge of
budin

foramen magnum

Ex-occipital (condylar)

Basi-occipital

Above the highest nuchal line the squamous part is developed in membrane, and is ossified from two centres about the second month of intrauterine life. The rest of bone is developed in cartilage, below the highest nuchal line the squamous part is developed from two centres which appear about the seventh week of intrauterine life. Union of the above takes place in the third month of intrauterine life. Each lateral part ossifies from a single centre during the eighth week of intrauterine life. The basilar portion is ossified from a single centre about the sixth week of intrauterine life. About the end of the second year, the squamous part unites with the lateral portions and by the sixth year the bone consists of a single piece.

Budin, P.C. , (1846-1907.)

THE SPHENOID BONE

The sphenoid is situated in the base of the skull and takes part in the formation of the floor, of the anterior, middle, and posterior cranial fossae, of the temporal and nasal fossae, and the orbital cavity. It is very irregular in shape and is described as consisting of a central part or body, two pairs of lateral expansions the greater and lesser wings and a pair of pterygoid processes which project downwards. It articulates with, - the occipital, temporal, frontal, ethmoid, parietal, sphenoidal turbinate, palatine, vomer, zygomatic and epipteric bone when present, occasionally with the maxilla. It has forty named processes and ridges, is traversed by sixteen foramina and forms part of the boundaries of ten others. It gives attachment to thirteen pairs of muscles, viz, - Lateral pterygoid, Medial pterygoid, Temporalis, Levator palpebrae superioris, Superior rectus, Inferior rectus, Lateral rectus, Medial rectus, Superior oblique, Tensor tympani, Tensor palati, Levator palati and the Superior constrictor muscle. The body, made by the union of two parts which represent the united pre and basi-sphenoid bones of other vertebrates. Its posterior part is rough and unites with the basi-occipital by synchondrosis before the age of twenty one, but after that age by synostosis. Above this is the upper part of the clivus or anterior wall of the posterior cranial fossa, raising forwards to the dorsum sellae. The sharp lateral margins of this portion slope downwards and outwards, and end in the sharp posterior petrosal process, which are joined by cartilage to the apices of the petrous temporalis. The upper surface present posteriorly the deep pituitary fossa or sella turcica, bounded behind by the square plate of bone the dorsum sellea, which ends on each side in a lateral tubercle, the posterior clinoid process, which gives attachment to the fixed margin of the tentorium cerbelli. On each side of the dorsum sellea is a notch for the passage of the abducent nerve. In the front of the fossa is an oval elevation, the tuberculum sellea, anterior to which is the transverse groove, sulcus chiamatis, which ends laterally in the optic foramina. This groove is bordered in front by a ridge, limbus sphenoidalis, from which a flat surface, jugum sphenoidale extends forwards, forming part of the floor of the anterior cranial fossa, ending anteriorly in the sharp ethmoidal spine which articulates with the posterior edge of the cribriform plate. The anterior boundary of the sella is completed laterally by two small eminences called the middle clinoid processes.

The lateral surfaces of the body are united with the great wings and with the medial pterygoid lamina. Above the attachment of each wing is a broad groove, the carotid sulcus, it is curved like the letter f ; it lodges the internal carotid artery and the cavernous sinus. The carotid sulcus is deepest at its posterior end where it is overhung medially by the petrosal process, and is limited laterally by a sharp margin called the lingula; the lingual is continued backwards to overlie the posterior opening of the pterygoid (Vidian), canal.

Three canals traverse the root of attachment of the great wing of the sphenoid along the outer side of the body. – the uppermost is the foramen for the maxillary division of the trigeminal, directly below the sphenoidal fissure; the second is the Vesalian foramen, an irregular vascular hole, often absent, transmitting a small vein; the third of Vidian canal traverses the line of attachment of the medial pterygoid plate to the side of the body, and transmits the artery and nerve of this canal. The side of the body of the sphenoid gives attachment above and in front to the lesser wing by two roots, the upper thin and flat, the lower thick and triangular; between these is the optic foramen which transmits the optic nerve and its coverings and the ophthalmic artery.

The anterior surface presents a median ridge, the sphenoidal crista, descending from the under surface of the ethmoid. The body of the sphenoid is seen in this aspect to be hollow, the cavity being divided by a median septum into two lateral parts, the sphenoidal sinuses. The septum, which is the backward continuation of the crest, is usually bent to one side. The opening of each side is bounded below and internally by a curved triangular bone, concave above, convex downwards and forwards, the sphenoidal tubinates or (ossicula bertini), which are originally separate bones in the adolescent skull. External to this opening of the sinuses is the vertical orbital lamella of the body of the sphenoid which joins the posterior edge of the orbital plate of ethmoid and presents below a palatine notch for the orbital process of the palatine bone. The lower surface forms the roof of the choanae and presents a median ridge, the sphenoidal rostrum which projects into a deep fissure between the anterior parts of the alae of the vomer.

On each side of the posterior part of the rostrum and immediately behind the apex of the sphenoidal concha of Bertini, a thin prominent lamella the vaginal process projects medially from the base of the medial pterygoid plate. Behind these the sphenoid becomes continuous with the basi-occipital (bone of Blumenbach). The lesser wings, the processes Ingrassia, are elongated and triangular, projecting from the side of the upper and anterior part of the body. They are flat above where they form part of the floor of the anterior cranial fossa. The front border is toothed to unite with the orbital plate of the frontal. The hinder edge is free and crescenteric, and corresponds to the Sylvian fissure in the brain, ending posteriorly and internally in a tubercle, the anterior clinoid process, which is directed towards the sella turcica, and often grooved on its inner side by the ophthalmic artery. The lower or orbital surface is smaller than the upper, and presents a sharp orbital ridge continuous with the front edge of the inferior root of the wing. The inferior surface forms the posterior part of the roof of the orbit and the upper boundary of the superior orbital fissure. This fissure transmits from the cranial to the orbital cavity, the oculomotor, trochlear, and abducent nerves, frontal, lacrimal and nasociliary branches of the ophthalmic division of the trigeminal nerve, and from the cavernous sympathetic filaments; and from the orbital cavity, the recurrent meningeal branch of the lacrimal artery and the ophthalmic veins. From the periosteum covering the orbital ridge and lesser wing, five orbital muscles arise. The apex of the wing is external, separated from the greater wing by a narrow slit, closed in the skull by the orbital process of the frontal. The greater wings are two strong processes which curve upwards and lateralwards from the sides of the body. Each presents four surfaces, - a concave superior forming the front part of the floor of the middle cranial fossa, a quadrate flat anterior or orbital making the chief part of the lateral wall of the orbit; a convex external or tempro-basilar, and a triangular frontal or sutural surface, which in the skull is covered by the orbital plate of the frontal. The superior surface is isolated by four edges – an internal, sharp edge, which forms the outer lip of the sphenoidal fissure; a superior which enters into suture with the frontal and parietal

Gido Guida (Vidus Vidius) (1500 – 1567). **Vesalius, A.** (1514 – 1564).
Blumenbach, J.F. (1752 – 1840). **Ingrassia, G.** (1510 – 1580). **Sylvius, F.** (1614 – 1672).

bones; an external concave, thicker behind which articulates with the squamous; and a posterior, straight edge joined by synchondrosis to the petrous. The external and posterior edges unite at the acute and back-directed spine of sphenoid, which is pierced by the foramen spinosum for the middle meningeal artery, and the recurrent meningeal branch of the mandibular division of the trigeminal nerve. The inner aspect is grooved by branches of the meningeal vessels. At its root is the round and Vesalian holes, behind and lateral to which is the foramen ovale, for the mandibular division of trigeminal, accessory meningeal artery, and occasionally the lesser superficial petrosal nerve. The thin plate of bone which bounds this behind is often pierced by a fine canalicus innominatus for the lesser superficial petrosal nerve. The spine of sphenoid is grooved on its medial surface for the chorda tympani nerve. The flat orbital surface, whose plane converges backwards to that of its fellow is bounded externally by a toothed edge crista zygomaticus, which joins the zygomatic, above by a sutural edge for the frontal, below its edge is rounded, and forms the hinder lip of the sphenomaxillary fissure, crista spheno-maxillaris, and internally its sharp edge forms the free margins of the sphenoidal fissure, crista orbitalis, a little in front of this is a tubercle for attachment of part of external rectus muscle. The temporo-basilar surface presents three parts, - temporal, infra-temporal and pterygoid. The horizontal infra-temporal crest limits the temporal area below, the temporal portion gives attachment to the temporalis muscle, is bounded in front by the crista zygomaticus; above it articulates with the parietal and frontal bones; behind, it is overlapped by the squamous temporal. The infra-temporal surface is bounded in front by the spheno-maxillary crest, and laterally articulates with the squamous; it gives attachment to the upper head of the lateral pterygoid muscle and at its hinder border presents the openings of the foramina ovale and spinosum. The lower surface of the spine is sometimes elongated downwards into a styloid process or spina angularis. Projecting downwards are the pterygoid plates, two on each side, medial and lateral. The medial pterygoid plate is the remains of the pterygoid bone and arises independently in the embryo. In the adult it forms the outer wall of the posterior nares, beginning above in a small process, the pterygoid tubercle, which is separated from the lingula and spheno-petrosal lamina above by the opening of the pterygoid canal. From this a more or less distinct edge is continued inwards towards the side of the rostrum, the margin then turns sharply forwards and projects as the vaginal process, which articulates anteriorly with the sphenoidal process of the palatine bone and medially with the ala of the vomer. The root of the vaginal process is often pierced by the pterygo-pharyngeal canal, which completed by the palatine bone, and transmits the pharyngeal nerve and artery. The root of the medial pterygoid plate is posteriorly depressed into a shallow scaphoid fossa, to which the Eustachian cartilage is attached, and from whose outer marginal ridge the tensor palati muscle arises. Where the ridge becomes confluent with the hinder margin of the medial pterygoid plate, a small process, the processes tubarius usually projects. The lower end of the medial pterygoid plate is prolonged backwards and outwards into a spur, the pterygoid hamalus, whose outer grooved surface forms a pulley for the tensor palate. Between the two pterygoid plates below is a triangular interspace into which the pyramidal process of the palatine bone is wedged. From the hamular process and lower half of the posterior border of the medial pterygoid plate, the superior constrictor of the pharynx arises. The lateral pterygoid plate projects further posteriorly, but not so low down as the medial. To its lateral surface is attached the lateral pterygoid muscle, to its medial surface the medial pterygoid. The surfaces are rough for the tendinous planes in these muscles. The fossa between the two pterygoid plates is the pterygoid fossa.

Eustachi, B. (1500 – 1574).

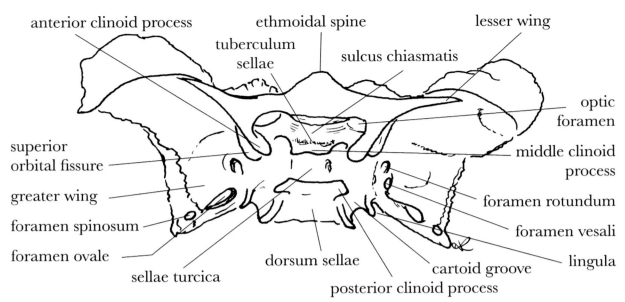

The sphenoid bone, superior aspect.

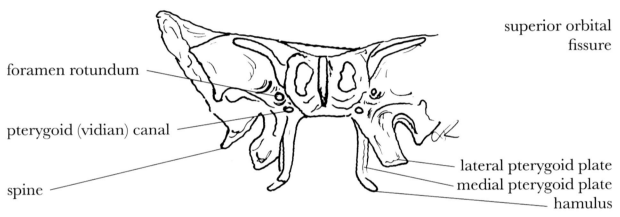

The sphenoid bone, anterior aspect.

THE SPHENOIDAL CONCHA OF BERTIN

The sphenoidal concha are two thin curved plates of bone, and are situated at the anterior and inferior part of the body of the sphenoid, where they close the sphenoidal sinuses. Each bone articulates with the rostrum of sphenoid, and ala of vomer, ethmoid, and orbital process of the palatine bone.

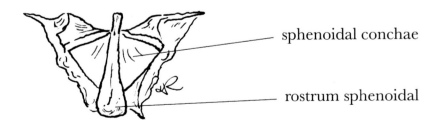

The sphenoidal conchae of Bertini.

Bertin. J. (1712 – 1781)

The sphenoid bone – until the eighth month of intrauterine life the body of the sphenoid consists of two parts – viz., one in front of the tuberculum sellae forming the presphenoid part, with which the lesser wings are continuous; the other comprising the sellae turcica and dorsum sellae, forming the post-sphenoid part, with which the greater wings and pterygoid processes are ossified, a deal is developed in cartilage.

Presphenoid has six centres.   Post-sphenoid has eight centres.

The presphenoid and postsphenoid parts fuse about the eighth month of foetal life, at birth the bone is in three parts; a central consisting of the body and lesser wings, and two lateral, each comprising a greater wing and a pterygoid process.   In the first year after birth the greater wings and body unite around the margins of the pterygoid canal, and the lesser wings extend medially above the anterior part of the body, and meet to form an elevated smooth surface called the jugum sphenoidale.

THE TEMPORAL BONE

The temporal bone is situated on each side of the lower part of the cranium. It contains the organs of hearing. It consists of four parts of very different origin, which at birth have united into a single bone. These are, - squamous; tympanic; petrous; and the styloid elements. The temporal bone articulates by suture with the occipital, parietal, sphenoid, zygomatic, and by a moveable joint with the mandible. Occasionally the squamous portion presents a process which articulates with the frontal.

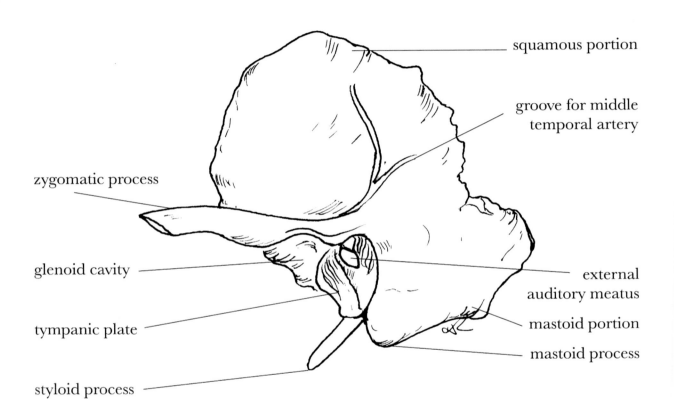

squamous portion

groove for middle
temporal artery

zygomatic process

glenoid cavity

tympanic plate

styloid process

external
auditory meatus

mastoid portion

mastoid process

The temporal bone, lateral surface.

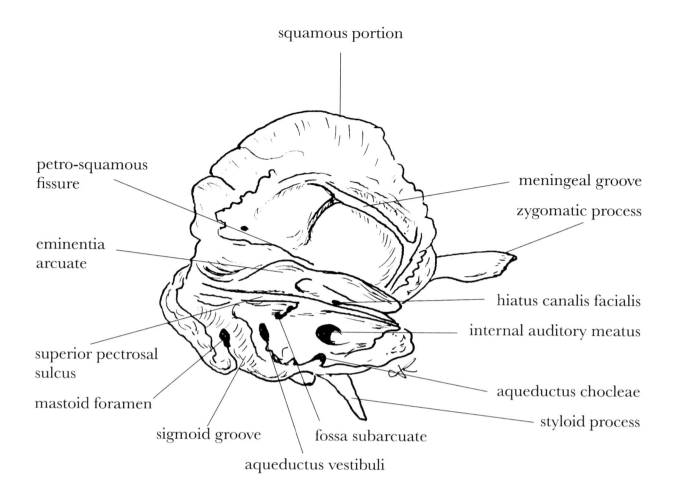

squamous portion

petro-squamous fissure

meningeal groove

zygomatic process

eminentia arcuate

hiatus canalis facialis

internal auditory meatus

superior pectrosal sulcus

mastoid foramen

aqueductus chocleae

styloid process

sigmoid groove

fossa subarcuate

aqueductus vestibuli

The temporal bone, medial aspect.

The temporal gives attachment to thirteen muscles, - squamous portion, temporalis, zygomatic process, masseter, mastoid process, sternocleidomastoid, splenius capitis, longissimus capitis, digastric posterior belly, posterior auricular, petrous portion, - levator palati, tensor tympani, stapedius.   styloid process, stylohyoid, styloglossus, stylopharyngeus.

The temporal bone is ossified from eight centres.   Squamous portion − ossified in membrane from one centre about the seventh − eighth week of intrauterine life. Petromastoid - from four centres which appear in the cartilaginous ear capsule about the fifth − sixth month of intrauterine life.   Tympanic ring − ossified in membrane from one centre, third month of intrauterine life.   Styloid process − (second visceral arch) from two centres.   One for proximal end (tympanohyal) before birth.   One for distal end (stylohyal) after birth.

Temporal bone

The squamous bone of the temporal is a thin plate; entering into the side wall of the middle cranial fossa. Its front edge is serrated to articulate with the hinder edge of the greater wing of the sphenoid, and its curved upper and thin hinder edges overlap the parietal in the squamous suture. Below it unites with to the petrous and tympanic parts. Its lateral flat surface forms part of the temporal fossa, giving origin to the **temporalis** muscle, and is faintly grooved for the posterior deep temporal vessels. The surface ends below at the **zygomatic arch**, which projects out as a self from its lower border, the surfaces of the process at its root being directed upwards and downwards; but as the zygoma turns forwards, it becomes twisted, and presents a smooth surface medially, a rougher surface laterally, a sharp edge (for the temporal fascia) upwards, a blunter edge for the **masseter** muscle downwards. From the root of the zygoma three ridges pass, one, the **post-auricular**, horizontally backwards, forming the hinder and lower end of the temporal crest as far as the parietal notch. Below this, as the bone descends to form the lateral wall of the mastoid process, is an irregular line, the remains of the obliterated suture between the petrous and squamous bones. A second **post-glenoid ridge** projects medially in front of the external auditory meatus, and joins the anterior border of the tympanic part. The third ridge or **tuberculum articulare** (eminentia articularis), it runs inwards and backwards, converging towards its fellow, the long axes, if prolonged, meeting in the mid-line at an angle of 135°; it forms the anterior boundary of the glenoid cavity for the mandible. The zygoma ends in front by articulating with the zygomatic (malar) bone in an irregular suture. Between the front edge of the tuberculum articulare and the sphenoidal margin is the triangular **infratemporal surface**, crossed by the external pterygoid muscle, separated from the temporal fossa by the **crista infratemporalis**. Where the former joins the zygoma, there is a **pre-genoid tubercle** for the attachment of the **temporomandibular ligament**. The glenoid cavity is bounded behind by a persistend suture between the tympanic and squamous parts of the bone, the **petrotympanic** (Glasserian) **fissure**, in which a minute rough line of petrous bone appears internally above and medial to glenoid cavity. Through this fissure the anterior tympanic artery, a branch of the maxillary, the anterior ligament of the malleus. Through the canal (**canal of Huguier**)

Between the tympanic and the ridge of petrous bone internally, the **chorda tympani nerve** escapes. The intracranial surface of the squamous part is smaller than the lateral, being overlapped by the lower edge of the parietal. It is deeply grooved by branches of the middle meningeal vessels, and is marked by depressions corresponding to the convolutions of the temporal lobe of the brain. A trace of the petrosquamosal suture often persists below as a faint fissure and is frequently seen in the adult bone.

The tympanic bone – The modified quadrate of lower vertebrates, partly replaced by a parostocic addition, bounds the external auditory meatus, and the tympanic cavity in front and below. Its external edge is rough and concave upwards, and forms the lower and front edge of the auditory passage. In front it is separated from the post –glenoid tubercle and glenoid cavity of the squamous by the petrotympanic fissure, extending inwards nearly as far as the sphenoidal notch. Posteriorly it is separated from the mastoid process by the **tympano-mastoid fissure**, through which **Arnold's** auricular branch of the vagus escapes.   Internally, this hinder edge fuses with the petrosal, being pierced, however, for the exit of the styloid process.   The tympanic part presents two surfaces, an antero-inferior, directed towards the glenoid cavity, from which it is separated by a lobe of the parotid gland; and a postero-superior, or tympanic which is concave towards the meatus and tympanic cavity, of which it forms the anterior wall.   The lower and hinder edge of the glenoid surface is prolonged downwards into sharp irregular ridge, the **vaginal process**, which starts from the lowest part of the lip of the auditory meatus, and extends forwards and inwards to end in front of the carotid foramen.   To this, the front of the fascial sheath of the carotid vessels is attached.

The styloid element is a slender cylindrical spur of variable length, which emerges through the most prominent part of the vaginal process.   It consists of two parts, a basal proximal part (**tympano-hyal**), embedded in the interspace between the tympanic and petrous parts and surrounded by its sheath (vagina processus styloidei), and a distal (**stylo-hyal**) part, to whose lateral edge is attached a fold of cervical fascia, the **stylomandibular ligament** tying it to the angle and hinder border of the ramus of the mandible.   Its lip is continued into a slender fibro-cartilage, the **stylohyoid ligament**, which is attached below to the lesser cornua of the hyoid bone. Behind and above the former ligament the **stylopharyngeus muscle** arises from the medial side of the base, and from the anterior and lateral side near the apex close to the latter ligament, arises the **styloglossus**.   The **stylohyoid** muscle arises between and behind these.

The petrous bone is an irregular four-sided pyramid, whose base extends backwards to the postero-external wall of the skull, where it forms the **mastoid region.**   Its truncated apex points forward and inwards to the **foramen lacerum**.   Its inferior surface is basilar, its anterior is tympanic, and the superior and posterior are intracranial. The base or mastoid region is externally rough and triangular, bounded above by the post-auricular ridge and the parieto-mastoid suture, behind by the ocipito-mastoid suture, and in front by the auditory meatus and the tympano-mastoid fissure.   It culminates in the **mastoid** process, whose irregular tip directed forwards and downwards, and into whose lateral surface the **sternomastoid, splenius capitis,** and **longissimus capitis** (trachelo-mastoid) are attached.   Internal to it is the groove for the **posterior belly** of **digastric**, which is separated by a ridge which widens backwards from a second groove for the **occipital artery**, close to the hinder end of which is the **mastoid** foramen transmitting a vein from the lateral transverse sinus, and the mastoid branch of the occipital artery to the mastoid aid cells and the dura mater, anastomosing with the middle meningeal artery.   From the front and upper part of the mastoid process arise the **posterior auriculae**, and a few fibres of the **occipito-frontalis** muscles.   The mastoid region on the inner surface of the skull is flattened and concave, completing the lateral part of the posterior cranial fossa, and deeply grooved where it joins the rest of the petrous bone by the downward and inward running deep sulcus for the **sigmoid sinus**.   Under the superficial layer of bone in the mastoid process, which is a descending lamella of the squamosal, are many large **mastoid cells,** which are arranged in three series, an anterior superior, very irregular, extending into the rest of the petrous bone, and communicating by a ragged passage with the back of the cavity of the tympanum, a middle set of large cells communicating with the anterior, and a third or apical set of small cells.   The first and second of these are lined with mucous membrane and contain air, the third series are usually marrow-holding.   The passage from the tympanum usually dilates under the down-growing lamella of the squamous part into an irregular cavity, the **mastoid antrum** (tympanic antrum).   The inferior of basilar surface of the petrous bone is irregular having its front and lateral part covered by the vaginal process of the tympanic, behind which it is pierced by the **stylomastoid foramen** for the exit of the **facial nerve**.   Internal to the styloid process is a smooth-walled pit, the **jugular fossa**, which forms the front part of the wall of the jugular foramen, and in which is contained a pouch-like dilation (**jugular bulb**) at the beginning of the internal jugular vein.   On the lateral wall of this fossa is a fine canal, the mastoid canaliculus, running laterally, for the auricular branch of the vagus (**Arnold's** nerve).   At its inner and front part is a small three-sided depression, the **aqueductus cochleae**, on the margin between the inferior and posterior surfaces, this rapidly narrows to a minute canal that transmits a prolongation of dura mater, and transmits a vein from the cochlea to join the internal jugular vein.   A sharp **carotid ridge** separates the front of the jugular fossa from the round opening of the **carotid canal** which lies in front, and which transmits the internal carotid artery.   Upon this ridge is the minute opening of the **tympanic canaliculus** for the **tympanic (Jacobson's)** branch of the glossopharyngeal nerve. The carotid canal ascends, then turns forwards and inwards, tunnelling the pertous bone to its apex, and finally runs into the upper part of the foramen lacerum.   Two minute **carotico-tympanic tubules** leave this canal and transmit minute nerves from the carotid plexus of sympathetics.   The apex of the bone is rough below, covered by the cartilage of the occipito-petrosal synchondrosis.   The posterior surface forms the antero-lateral wall of the posterior cranial fossa.   It is grooved along its inner border by the inferior petrosal sinus, lateral to which is an outward-directed orifice, the **internal auditory meatus**, which, at a depth of about 8mm. ends in the **reniform fossa**, pierced above by the **aqueductus Fallopi** for the facial nerve, and by a group of holes below, **macula cribrosa**, for the auditory nerve.   Along the upper margin, between the meatus and the superior surface, is a groove for the superior petrosal sinus, below which, on a plane behind the meatus is an irregular opening, the **floccular fossa** or **hiatus subarcuatus**, very large in the young bone though often obliterated in the adult, which burrows under the semicircular canal.

Behind and below this is the slit-like **aqueductus vestibule** which contains the ductus endolymphaticus together with a small artery and vein.   The aqueduct of Fallopius (canalis facialis) runs at first laterally then turns backwards and finally descends to the **stylomastoid foramen**   The superior surface forms the back part of the floor of the middle cranial fossa, and by its apex is joined to the petrosal process of the sphenoid, in front of which it is often grooved by the upturning carotid artery.   Close to the apex is a pit for the trigeminal (Gasserian) ganglion, in front of which is the ragged foramen lacerum from whose margin two fine grooves run backwards and laterally, leading to two small holes, the hinder of which for the hiatus Fallopii for the greater superficial petrosal nerve, the foremost is for the lesser superficial petrosal.   Behind and lateral to these is an oblique eminence, the **eminentia arcuata** or jugum petrosum, over the superior semicircular canal, directly laterally to which the bone is thin and irregular, roofing in the tympanic cavity and named the **tegmen tympani**.   This is frequently divided by a fissure into an outer or cuneiform portion, and an inner or **tegmen proprium**. At the posterior part of this surface there are small irregular vascular holes transmitting minute veins into the lateral (transverse) sinus. The anterior or tympanic surface is shown by removing the tympanic bone and the cartilage of the Eustachian tube, and forms the inner wall of the tympanic cavity. Laterally it forms part of the wall of the external meatus as far as the annulus for the attachment of the tympanic membrane, next it is pierced by an irregular **mastoid antrum** above, which communicates with the mastoid air cells. Below this the **fenestra ovalis** or opening into the vestibule, placed over a convex projection or **promontory** grooved for the nerves from the different tympanic canals; still lower and a little farther back is a three-sided **fenestra rotunda** opening into the cochlea; behind this is a small hollow process, the **pyramid**, juts forwards, whose base is traversed by a hole which leads into the aqueduct Fallopius. In front and above the fenestra ovalis a thin curved plate of bone, the **processus cochleariformis**, projects backwards and upwards as a partition, subdividing the space which exists between the petrous bone and the overlying layer of the tympanic bone into two tubes, which extend from the hindmost part of the spheno-petrosal sulcus into the cavity of the tympanum. The lower of these is the **Eustachian tube,** communicating between the pharynx and the tympanium; the upper is the canal for the **tensor tympani**. The remaining anterior portion of this surface, internal to the tympanic bone gives attachment to the cartilage of the Eustachian tube. The rough irregular line of junction between the inferior and internal aspects of the petrous bone gives origin to the **levator palati** and **tensor palate** muscles and to the pharyngeal aponeurosis (pharyngo-basilar fascia). Other structural details of the petrous bone are described in connection with the anatomy of the ear. Small ossicles (the **bones of Riolan**) are frequently developed along the petro-occipital suture.

Riolan, J. The younger (1580 – 1657)

THE ETHMOID BONE

This bone is of delicate texture, being situated at the anterior part of the floor of the anterior cranial fossa; projecting downwards between the orbital plates of the frontal bone. It enters into the formation of the orbital and nasal fossae; it is cuboidal in shape and its extreme lightness and delicacy is due to the arrangement of very thin plates of bone surrounding irregular spaces known as the ethmoidal air sinuses. It consists of four parts, - horizontal or cribriform plate, lateral masses, and perpendicular plate. It articulates with the frontal palatines, sphenoidal, nasals, vomer, inferior concha, lacrimal bones, and maxilla.

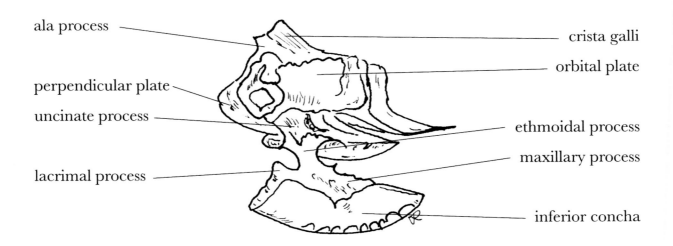

ala process

crista galli

orbital plate

perpendicular plate

uncinate process

ethmoidal process

maxillary process

lacrimal process

inferior concha

The ethmoid and inferior concha, left side.

The inferior concha, is a slender scroll-like lamina, attached by its upper margin to the lateral wall of the nasal fossa, and suspended into the cavity in such a way as to separate the middle from the inferior meatus. It articulates with the maxilla, lacrimal, palatine and ethmoid.

The ethmoid is ossified in the cartilaginous nasal capsule from three centres. One for the perpendicular plate during first year. Two centres, one for each labyrinth during fourth and fifth months of intrauterine life.

The inferior concha is ossified from one centre in the fifth month of intrauterine life.

Robson's Approach To Anatomy

THE VOMER

Is a single median vertical plate which forms the posterior and inferior part of the nasal septum.   It is thin and irregularly quadrilateral in shape, and is usually bent somewhat to one side, though the deflection rarely involves the posterior margin.   It is traversed by a narrow but well marked groove which lodges the naso-palatine nerve.

The vomer articulates with two maxillae, two palatine bones, the ethmoid and sphenoid and forms part of two pairs of foramina, the posterior nares, and the anterior palatine.

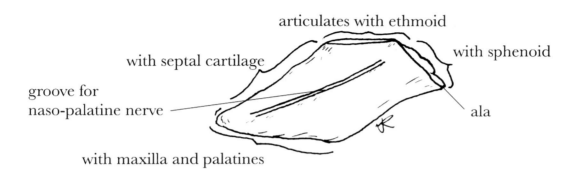

The vomer, left lateral surface.

The vomer is ossified in membrane from two centres about the eighth week of intrauterine life.

THE PALATINE BONE

The palatine bone is rectangular in shape, and forms the posterior part of the hard palate, the lateral wall of the nasal fossa, between the maxilla and medial pterygoid plate, and by its orbital process the posterior part of the floor of the orbit. It articulates with six bones, - viz, sphenoid, maxilla, vomer, inferior nasal concha, and ethmoid. The palatine bone – is ossified in membrane from one centre about the eighth week of intrauterine life. It gives attachment to five muscles, - viz, medial pterygoid, tensor palate, musculus uvulae, and palatopharyngeus.

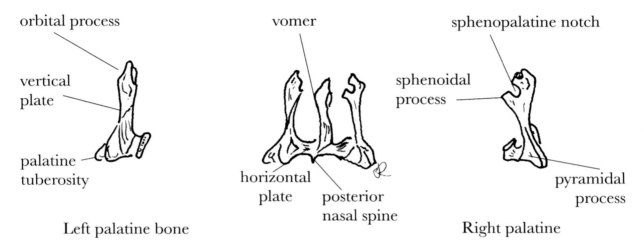

orbital process

vomer

sphenopalatine notch

vertical plate

sphenoidal process

palatine tuberosity

horizontal plate   posterior nasal spine

pyramidal process

Left palatine bone

Right palatine

THE NASAL BONES

The nasal bones are two contiguous, oblong bones whose shape determines the form of the nose. They are situated at the upper part of the facial skeleton. Each bone articulates with the maxillae, frontal and ethmoid, and its fellow of the opposite side. Their facial surface present a nasal foramen, for a nasal tributary of the facial vein. They are grooved on their internal surface for the anterior ethmoidal nerve.

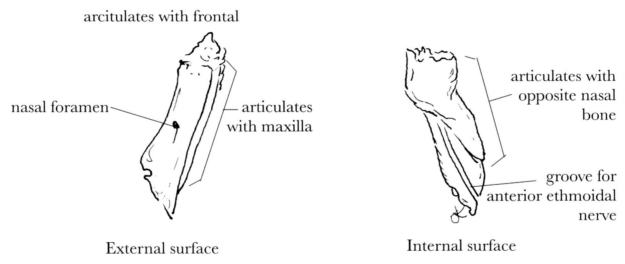

arcitulates with frontal

nasal foramen

articulates with maxilla

articulates with opposite nasal bone

groove for anterior ethmoidal nerve

External surface

Internal surface

The nasal bone is ossified in membrane at the beginning of the third month of intrauterine life.

THE LACRIMAL BONE

The lacrimal bone is small, delicate and quadrilateral in shape, is situated at the anterior part of the medial wall of the orbit, it is the smallest of the facial bones. It articulates with the ethmoid, frontal, maxilla, and inferior concha, and gives attachment to one muscle, the lacrimal part of orbicularis oculi.

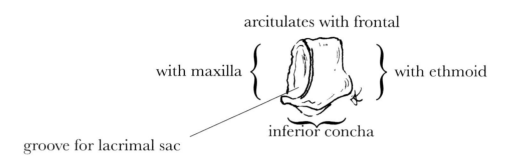

The lacrimal bone is ossified in membrane about the twelfth week of intrauterine life.

THE ZYGOMATIC (MALAR) BONE

The zygomatic bone forms the prominence known as the cheek, it joins the zygomatic process of the temporal with the maxilla. It is quadrilateral in shape with its angles directed vertically and horizontally. It articulates with the frontal, maxilla, sphenoid and temporal; and gives attachment to four muscles, - levator labii superioris, zygomaticus major, zygomaticus minor, and masseter.

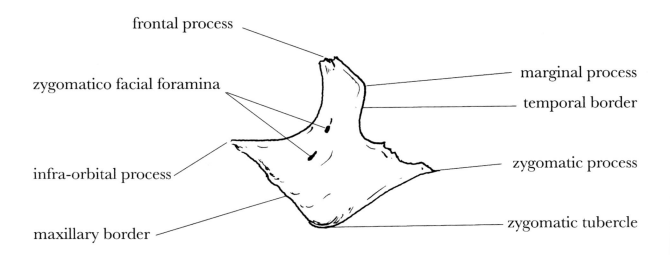

The zygomatic bone, left lateral surface.

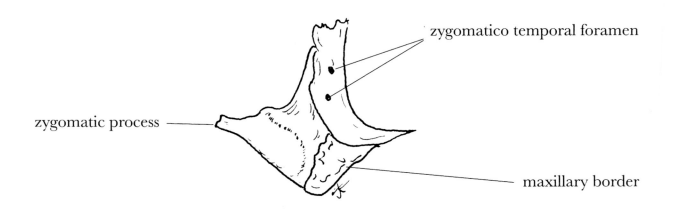

The zygomatic bone, left lateral surface.

The zygomatic bone is ossified in membrane from one centre about the eighth week of intrauterine life.

THE MAXILLA

The maxilla is one of the most important bones of the face. It supports the upper teeth and takes part in the formation of the orbit, the hard palate, and the nasal fossa. It is divided into a body which contains the maxillary sinus, four processes, of which two – the frontal and zygomatic belong to the upper part, while the palatal and alveolar to the lower part of the bone. It articulates with nine bones, - viz, frontal, nasal, lacrimal, ethmoid, palatine, vomer, zygomatic, inferior nasal concha, and its fellow of the opposite side. Occasionally it articulates with the great wing of sphenoid and its pterygoid process.

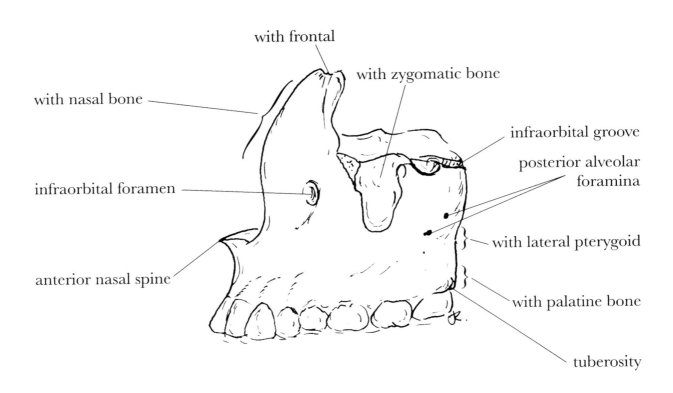

The maxilla, left lateral surface.

The maxilla gives attachment to nine muscles, - viz, orbicularis oculi, inferior oblique, levator labii superioris alaeque nasi, levator labii superioris, levator anguli oris, nasalis, transverse (compressor naris) part, alar part, (dilator naris), depressor septi, masseter, and buccinators.

It is ossified in membrane from two principal centres, one for the maxilla proper, and one for the os incisivum at about the end of the sixth week of intrauterine life.

THE MANDIBLE

The mandible is the largest and strongest bone of the face. It supports the mandibular teeth, and by means of a pair of condyles articulates at the mandibular fossa of the temporal bones (tempromandibular joint). It consists of a horizontal portion, the body – strongly curved, so as to somewhat resemble a horseshoe, from the ends of which two perpendicular portions or rami ascend almost at right angles. It gives attachment to fourteen pairs of muscles, - viz, depressor labi inferioris, depressor anguli oris, platysma, buccinators, masseter, geniohyoid, genioglossus, mylohoid, digastric anterior belly, superior constrictor, temporalis, lateral pterygoid, medial pterygoid, and mentalis.

The mandible is ossified in the fibrous membrane covering the outer surface of Meckel's cartilage. Each half of the mandible is ossified from one centre which appears near the mental formamen about the sixth week of intrauterine life, just after the primary centres for the clavicle.

Meckel, J.F.II (The younger) (1781 – 1833)

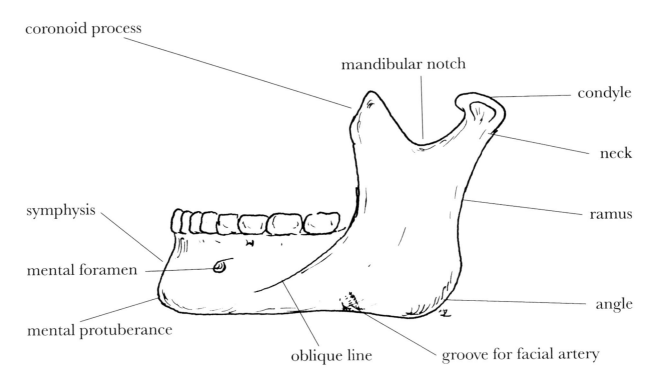

coronoid process

mandibular notch

condyle

neck

symphysis

ramus

mental foramen

mental protuberance

angle

oblique line

groove for facial artery

Left half of the mandible, lateral aspect.

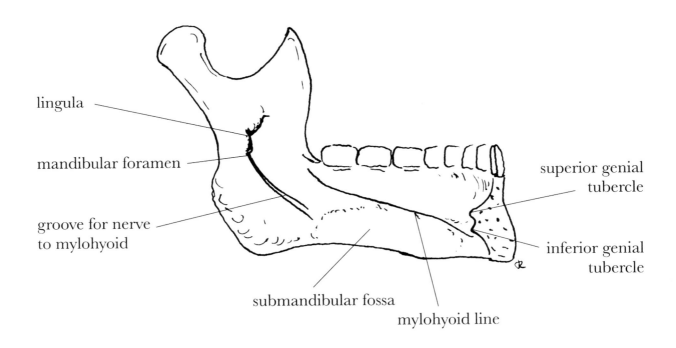

lingula

mandibular foramen

superior genial tubercle

groove for nerve to mylohyoid

inferior genial tubercle

submandibular fossa

mylohyoid line

Left half of the mandible, medial aspect.

THE HYOID BONE

The hyoid or os linguae is situated in the anterior part of the neck between the mandible above, and the thyroid cartilage below. It supports the tongue and gives attachment to numerous muscles. The hyoid is suspended from the tips of the styloid process of the temporal bones, by two slender ligaments, the stylohoids, and is divisible into a body, and two processes, the greater and lesser cornua.

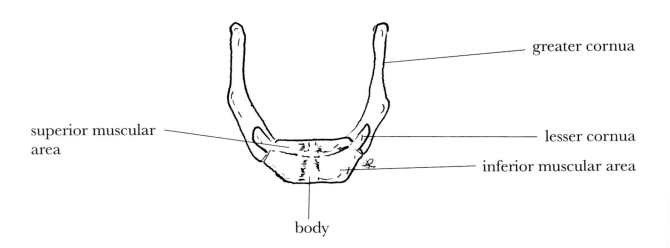

The hyoid bone.

The hyoid gives attachment to ten pairs of muscles:- geniohyoid, geniohyoglossus, chondroglossus, hyoglossus, omohoid superior belly, thyrohyoid, sternohyoid, mylohyoid, stylohyoid, digastric intermediate tendon, and middle constrictor. It is developed from the cartilages of the second and third visceral arches. The lesser cornua from the second, and the greater from the third, and the body from the fused ventral ends of both. It is ossified from six centres, a pair for the body and one for each cornua. Ossification commences in the greater cornua towards the end of intrauterine life, in the body before or shortly after and the lesser cornua during the first or second year.

THE AUDITORY OSSICLES

These three small bones are contained in the upper part of the tympanic cavity together they form a moveable chain, connecting the tympanic membrane to the fenestra vestibule. The malleus is attached to the tympanic membrane, and the base of the stapes to the circumference of the fenestra vestibuli, the incus is interposed between articulating with the malleus and stapes.

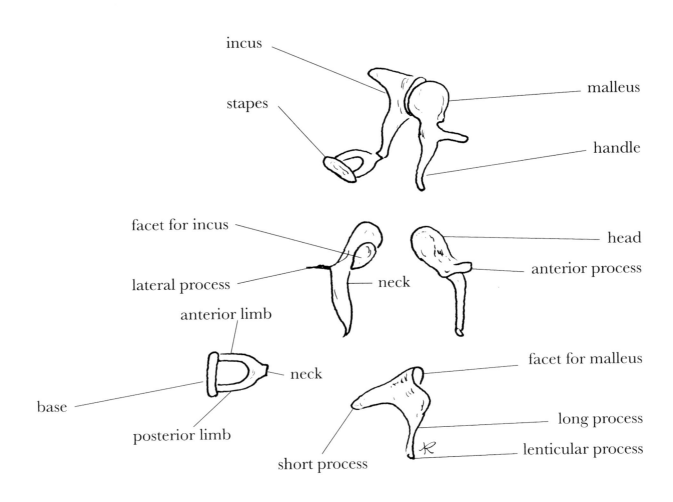

The malleus gives attachment to two muscles, tensor tympani and laxator tympani. The incus has no muscular attachments and the stapes has one muscle inserted into it, the stapedius. The malleus and incus are ossified from the dorsal end of the first arch cartilage Meckel's. The stapes is ossified from the dorsal end of the second arch cartilage Reichert's.

Meckel, J.F. II (1781 – 1833)

Reichert, K.B. (1811 – 1883)

THE SKULL AS A WHOLE

The skull formed by the union of the cranial and facial bones. When considered as a whole is bilaterally symmetrical, and is divisible into six regions; a superior or (**norma verticalis**), a posterior or (**norma occipitalis**), an anterior or (**norma facialis**), an inferior base or (**norma basilaris**), and two lateral or (**norma lateralis**). The bones of the cranium and face are connected to each other by means of sutures. The cranial sutures are divided into three sets. 1) Those of the vertex. 2) Those of the side of the skull. 3) Those of the base.

1) Sutures of the vertex are three in number, a) The sagittal (arrow) is situated between the two parietals, and extends from the bregma to the lambda. b) The coronal lies between the frontal and parietals, and extends from pterion to pterior. c) The lambdoid is formed by the parietals and interparietal portion of the occipital bone. It extends from the asterion to asterion. Occasionally there is found in some skulls a metopic suture, extending just above the glabella and involves the whole length of the frontal bone. The more important regions are: - The bregma, which indicates the situation of the anterior fontanelle, and marks the confluence of the coronal, sagittal, and when present the metopic sutures. The lambda, where the sagittal enters the lamboid suture, it marks the position of the posterior fontanelle. The obelion, a little anterior to the lambda, is usually indicated by a median or two lateral foramina.

2) Those of the side of the skull are three in number. a) Spheno-parietal. b) Squamo-parietal. c) Masto-parietal. They are subdivisions of a single suture formed between the lower border of the sphenoid, parietal and temporal bones, which extends from the inferior end of the lambdoid suture behind and coronal suture in front.

3) Of the base. a) The basilar suture, formed at the junction of the basilar process of the occipital bone and body of sphenoid. There is between the lateral end of the basilar suture and termination of the lambdoid an irregular suture which exists that is subdivided into two parts, a medial – between the union of the petrous temporal with the occipital, the petro-occipital suture. A lateral at the junction of the mastoid of temporal and occipital, the masto-occipital suture.

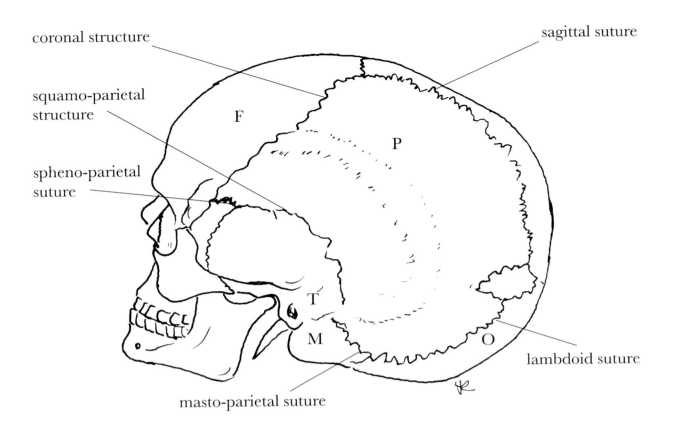

coronal structure

squamo-parietal structure

spheno-parietal suture

sagittal suture

lambdoid suture

masto-parietal suture

| F | Frontal Bone | P | Parietal bone | T | Temporal bone |
| M | Mastoid process | O | Occipital bone | | |

The cranial sutures.

THE EXTERIOR OF THE SKULL

1) The superior aspect (**norma verticalis**) is oval with the broader end posteriorly. 2) Viewed from behind (**norma occipitalis**) the skull appears somewhat pentagonal with rounded angles and sides; the upper medial angle is at the sagittal suture, the upper lateral at the parietal eminences, between these is the rounded upper part of the parietal bone. The inferior lateral angles are the mastoid processes. Between the mastoid processes is an irregular intermastoid basal line forming the fifth side. About 7.5cm below the mid-point of the lambdoid suture as seen in this aspect is a median occipital protuberance, or union, the occipital crest and the three pairs of nuchal lines. 3) The full-face view of the skull (**norma facialis**) is limited above by the bulge of the parietal bones behind the coronal suture and by the front of the squamous temporal on each side. Below the supercilliary ridges are the orbits, each of which is a conical cavity whose axis converges posteriorly to that of its fellow, so that, if prolonged, they would meet under the bregma.

The nasal region, between and below the orbits is closed in above by the nasal bones which unite medially in the internasal suture. It is open below at the anterior nares, whose long axis is vertical. The aperture is bounded above by the lower edges of the nasal bones, below by the anterior nasal narial lip of the maxilla, in the middle of which the anterior nasal spine projects; on each side is the sharp nasal margin of the maxilla. Within the opening is seen medially the anterior edge of the bony septum, consisting of the nasal lamella of the ethmoid above, and the vomer below. On each side of this septum is the nasal fossa. Between the edge of the anterior nares above and the sockets of the front teeth below, is a shallow pit on each side, bounded externally by the projecting canine socket, outside which is the canine fossa. Between this depression and the orbital brim is the infraorbital foramen.

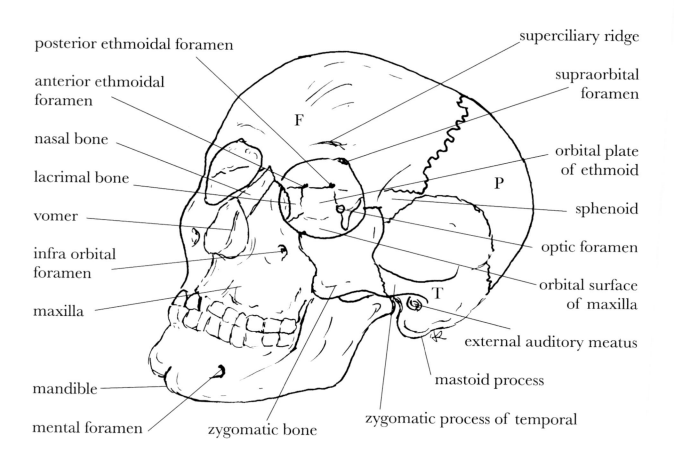

F Frontal Bone   P Parietal bone   T Temporal bone

The anterior and lateral regions of the skull.

4) Inferior base(**norma basilaris**) is very irregular and extends from the incisor teeth to the external occipital protuberance, and is bounded on each side by the alveolar arch of maxilla, zygomatic and zygomatic process of temporal, and the superior nuchal line of the occipital bone.   It is very uneven, and excluding the mandible is divisible into three regions; a) anterior, b) middle or subcranial, c) posterior or suboccipital.   a) The anterior region consists of the hard palate, the alveolar arch, and the posterior nares.   When the skull is inverted, the hard palate is at a higher level than the rest, and is bounded anteriorly and laterally by the alveolar ridges containing the teeth.   The bones appearing in the intermediate space are the pre-maxillary and the palatine processes of the maxillae, and the horizontal plates of the palatine bone.   Near the posterior margin is the ridge for the fibrous expansion of the tensor palati muscle. b) the middle or subcranial region is separated from the infratemporal fossa by a line drawn from the posterior margin of the external pterygoid plate to the spine of the sphenoid.   It is formed by the under surface of the basilar process of the occipital bone and body of sphenoid, the petrous part of the temporal bone, a small part of squamous temporal, the posterior part great wind of sphenoid, and the condylar processes of the occipital bone. c) The posterior or sub-occipital region is largely formed by the squamous portion of the occipital bone with its ridges and muscular areas.   Externally a small part of the mastoid process of the temporal bone is seen, pierced by a foramen of variable size, the mastoid foramen, which transmits a vein from the lateral sinus and meningeal branch of the occipital artery.   5) The lateral (**norma lateralis**) is somewhat triangular in shape, being bounded above by a line extending from the zygomatic process of the frontal, along the temporal crest, to the lateral part of the superior nuchal line of the occipital bone.   This forms the base of the triangle.   The two sides are represented by lines drawn from the extremities of the base to the angle of the mandible.   It is divisible into two parts, one anterior, the other posterior to the eminentia articularis.   The posterior part presents a horizontal line from behind forwards, the mastoid process and foramen, the external auditory meatus, the centre of which is known as the auricular point, the mandibular fossa, and the condyle of the mandible.   In the anterior part there are three fossae, 1) temporal, 2) infra-temporal, 3) spheno-maxillary.

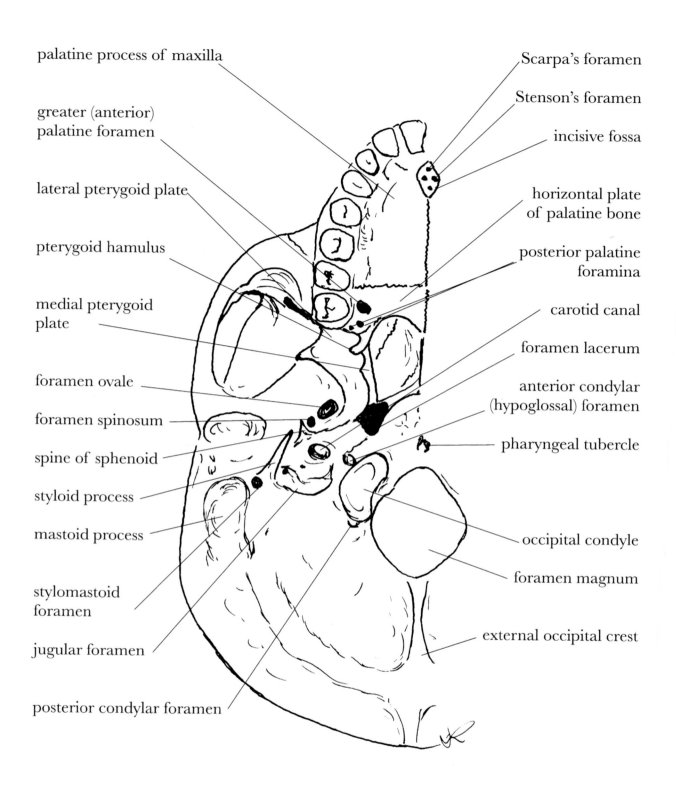

palatine process of maxilla

greater (anterior)
palatine foramen

lateral pterygoid plate

pterygoid hamulus

medial pterygoid
plate

foramen ovale

foramen spinosum

spine of sphenoid

styloid process

mastoid process

stylomastoid
foramen

jugular foramen

posterior condylar foramen

Scarpa's foramen

Stenson's foramen

incisive fossa

horizontal plate
of palatine bone

posterior palatine
foramina

carotid canal

foramen lacerum

anterior condylar
(hypoglossal) foramen

pharyngeal tubercle

occipital condyle

foramen magnum

external occipital crest

The base of the skull.

Scarpa, A. (1747 – 1832)

Stenson, N. (1638 – 1686)

Robson's Approach To Anatomy

1) **The temporal fossa** is bounded above and posteriorly by the temporal ridge, anteriorly by the frontal, zygomatic, and great wing of sphenoid, and laterally by the zygomatic arch.   2) **The infra-temporal fossa**, is bounded anteriorly by the medial surface of the zygomatic bone, and by the medial portion of the upper part posterior surface of the maxilla, on which are the posterior superior alveolar foramina; posteriorly by the posterior border of the lateral pterygoid plate, spine of sphenoid, and eminentia articularis, above by the infra temporal ridge, small part of squamous, part of temporal, the great wing of the sphenoid perforated by foramen ovale and foramen spinosum, inferiorly by the alveolar border of maxilla; laterally by the ramus of the mandible and the zygoma formed by the zygomatic and temporal bones; medially by the lateral pterygoid plate, a line from which to the spine of the sphenoid separates the infra temporal fossa from the base of the skull.   3) **The spheno-maxillary** is horizontal in position and lies between the maxilla, and great wing of sphenoid.   Through the fissure the orbit communicates with the pterygo-palatine (spheno-maxillary), infra-temporal and temporal fossa.   It transmits the infra orbital nerve, and vessels, the zygomatic nerve, ascending branches from the sphenopalatine ganglion, and communicating vein from the infra orbital to the pterygoid venous plexus.   b) **The pterygo-palatine** (pterygo-maxillary) fissure, forms a right angle with the spheno-maxillary fissure, and is situated between the maxilla and anterior border of pterygoid process of the sphenoid. It transmits branches of maxillary artery and veins to and from the pterygo-palatine fossa.   c) **The pterygo-palatine** (Spheno-maxillary) fossa, situated at the junction of the spheno-maxillary with the ptergo-palatine fissure.   It is bounded anteriorly by the medial portion of the upper part of the posterior surface of the maxilla; behind by root of the pterygoid process and the lower part of the anterior surface of the greater wing of the sphenoid, medially by the perpendicular plate upper part of the palatine bone with its orbital and sphenoidal processes, above by the under surface of the body of the sphenoid.   Including the spheno-palatine foramen six foramina open into the fossa. Of these, three are on the posterior wall; enumerated from without inwards, and from above downwards they are the foramen rotundum, the pterygoid (Vidian) canal, and the pharyngeal (pterygo-palatine) canal.   The apex of the pyramid leads below into the palatine canal, above it communicates with the orbit through the medial or posterior part of the infra orbital fissure.   The fossa contains the sphenopalatine ganglion, the maxillary nerve, and the terminal part of the maxillary artery and the various foramina and canals in relation with the fossa serve for the transmission of the numerous branches which these vessels and nerves give off.

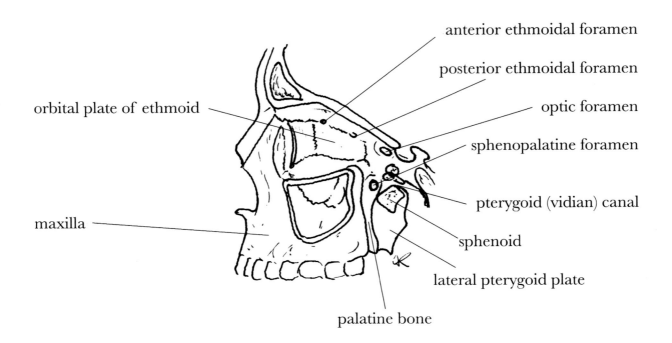

The pterygo-palatine fossa.

THE INTERIOR OF THE CRANIUM

The floor of the cranial cavity presents three irregular depressions called the anterior, middle and posterior fossa.

The anterior cranial fossa is bounded in front by the frontal bone; the floor is formed by the horizontal (orbital) parts of the frontal, the cribriform plate of ethmoid, the anterior part of body of sphenoid bone, and the lesser wings.

The middle cranial fossa is bounded in front by the posterior borders lesser wings of sphenoid, anterior clinoid processes and the anterior margin of sulcus chiamatis, behind by the superior borders of petrous parts of temporal bones, and the dorsum sellae, laterally by the squamous temporal, the frontal angles of parietal bones, and the greater wings of sphenoid.

The posterior cranial fossa is the largest and deepest of the cranial fossa, it is bounded in front by the dorsum sellae, posterior part of body of sphenoid and basilar part of occipital; behind by the lower part of squamous temporal, on each side by

Petrous and mastoid parts of temporal bones, lateral part of occipital bone, and above by a small part of the mastoid angle of the parietal bone.

The interior of the skull.

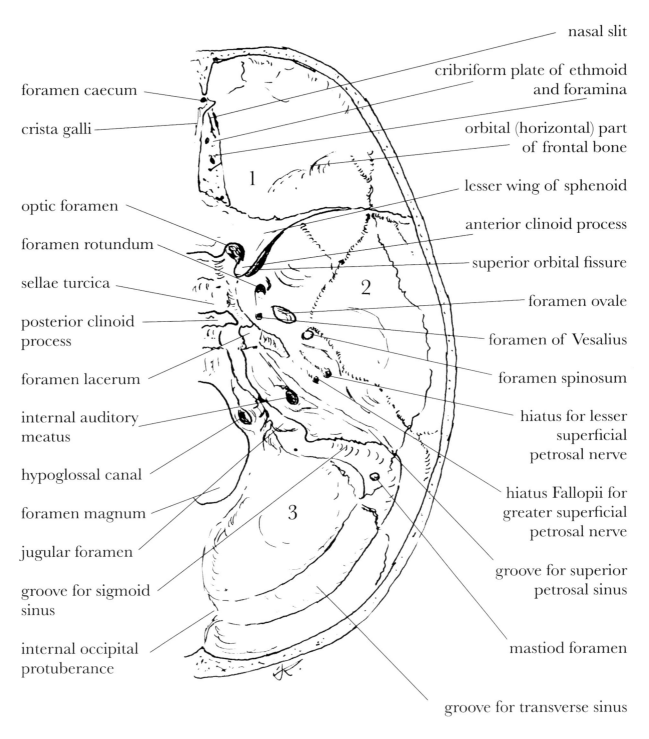

foramen caecum

crista galli

optic foramen

foramen rotundum

sellae turcica

posterior clinoid
process

foramen lacerum

internal auditory
meatus

hypoglossal canal

foramen magnum

jugular foramen

groove for sigmoid
sinus

internal occipital
protuberance

nasal slit

cribriform plate of ethmoid
and foramina

orbital (horizontal) part
of frontal bone

lesser wing of sphenoid

anterior clinoid process

superior orbital fissure

foramen ovale

foramen of Vesalius

foramen spinosum

hiatus for lesser
superficial
petrosal nerve

hiatus Fallopii for
greater superficial
petrosal nerve

groove for superior
petrosal sinus

mastiod foramen

groove for transverse sinus

1. Anterior cranial fossa   2. Middle cranial fossa.   3. Posterior cranial fossa.

Fallopio, G. (1523 – 1563)

Vesalius, A. (1514 – 1564)

THE FORAMINA OF THE SKULL

1) The base (**norma basilaris**) a) The incisive fossa, contains four small canals; two small orifices, foramina of scarpa – superior for left nasopalatine nerve, inferior for right masopalatine nerve, situated one behind the other, and two larger, the foramina of Stenson for incisive branches of the sphenopalatine artery. b) The greater palatine foramen, transmits the greater (anterior) palatine nerve, and vessels. c) The lesser palatine foramina, transmits the middle and posterior palatine nerves. d) The pterygoid (Vidian) canal, transmits the nerve of pterygoid canal, and a branch of the internal carotid artery, and a branch from the third part of maxillary. e) Hypoglossal (anterior condylar) canal, transmits the hypoglossal nerve, filaments of C. 1 nerve, and a meningeal branch of ascending pharyngeal artery. f) The foramen magnum, lower end of medulla oblongata, and its three membranes, cerebro-spinal fluid, vertebral artery, anterior and posterior spinal arteries, the spinal accessory nerve, apical ligament of the odontoid process, alar ligaments, menbrana tectoria. g) The carotid canal, transmits the internal carotid artery, internal carotid nerve from superior cervical ganglion (sympathetics). h) The jugular foramen, transmits the glossopharyngeal, vagus, accessory nerves, inferior petrosal sinus, sigmoid sinus, meningeal branch of occipital and ascending pharyngeal arteries. i) The jugular fossa, in bony ridge dividing fossa from carotid canal is the tympanic canaliculus for the tympanic branch of the glossopharyngeal, (Jacobson's nerve). In the lateral part of jugular fossa is the mastoid canaliculus for the auricular branch of the vagus (Arnold's nerve and foramen).

jugular fossa

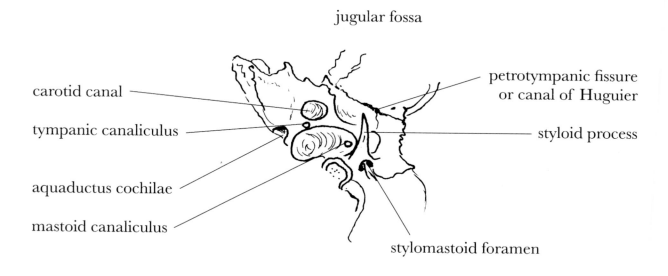

carotid canal

petrotympanic fissure or canal of Huguier

tympanic canaliculus

styloid process

aquaductus cochilae

mastoid canaliculus

stylomastoid foramen

Jugular fossa, left temporal bone.

Arnold, F. (1803 – 1890)
Jacobson, L. L. (1783 – 1843)
Huguier, P.C. (1804-1873)

Robson's Approach To Anatomy

J) The stylomastoid foramen, transmits the facial nerve, and the stylomastoid branch of the posterior auricular artery. k) The mastoid foramen, transmits the mastoid emissary vein. l) The foramen lacerum is filled in by a fibrocartilaginous plate, on the upper surface rest the internal carotid artery, surrounded by the carotid plexus of sympathetic nerves, the nerve of the pterygoid canal, and a branch of the ascending pharyngeal artery pierce the fibrocartilage. m) Posterior condylar foramen, transmits emissary vein, and meningeal branch of occipital artery. n) Palatovaginal canal, transmits the pharyngeal branch of the sphenopalatine ganglion.

The anterior (**norma facialis**) a) Supra-orbital notch or foramen, transmits the supra orbital nerve and vessels. b) Infra orbital foramen, transmits the infra orbital nerve and vessels. c) Mental foramen, transmits the mental nerve and vessels. d) Zygomaticotemporal foramen, transmits the zygomaticotemporal nerve. e) Zygomaticofacial foramen, transmits the zygomaticofacial nerve.

The lateral (**norma lateralis**) a) Pterygopalatine fossa, contains the maxillary nerve, third part of maxillary artery, and the sphenopalatine (Meckel) ganglion. b) Posterior alveolar canals, transmits the posterior superior alveolar nerves and vessels. c) Pterygopalatine (palatine) canal, transmits the palatine nerves and vessels. d) Sphenopaltine foramen, transmits the long and short nasopalatine nerves and sphenopalatine vessels. e) Inferior orbital fissure, transmits the maxillary nerve, zygomatic branch, infraorbtial vessels, orbital branch of sphenopalatine ganglion, and veins which connect the inferior ophthalmic vein with the pterygoid venous plexus.

The interior of the skull a) Foramen caecum, transmits a vein from the nose to superior sagittal sinus. Nasal slit of cribriform plate, transmits the nasocilliary nerve. c) Foramina in cribriform plate, transmits filaments of olfactory nerves. d) Optic foramen, transmits the optic nerve and its meninges, and the ophthalmic artery. e) Superior orbital fissure, transmits the abducent, trochlear, oculomotor, and lacrimal, frontal and nasocilliary branches of ophthalmic division of trigeminal nerve, and the superior ophthalmic vein. f) Foramen rotundum, transmits the maxillary division of trigeminal nerve.

g) Foramen ovale, transmits the mandibular division of trigeminal nerve, accessory meningeal artery, occasionally the lesser superficial petrosal nerve. h) Canaliculis innominatus when present transmits the lesser superficial petrosal nerve. i) Foramen of Vesalius (sphenoidal emissary foramen), transmits an emissary vein from the cavernous sinus to pterygoid venous lexus. j) Foramen spinosum, transmits the middle meningeal artery and vein, nervous spinosus, (recurrent meningeal branch of mandibular division of trigeminal). k) Hiatus, for lesser superficial petrosal nerve. l) Hiatus fallopii, for greater superficial petrosal nerve. m) Internal auditory meatus, for the facial nerve, nervus intermedius, vestibulocochlear nerve, and the labyrinthine artery.

Medial wall of orbit a) Anterior ethmoidal foramen, transmits the anterior ethmoidal nerve. b) Posterior ethmoidal foramen, transmits the posterior ethmoidal nerve.

Meckel, J. (1714 – 1774).

Medical Personalities mentioned throughout the text, each with a short biographical note.

Arnold, Friedrich. 1803-1890.
Professor of Anatomy at Zürich 1835, Freiburg 1840, then Tübingen 1845 and finally Heidleburg 1852.
Arnold's Nerve; Auricular branch of the vagus nerve.
Arnold's Ganglion; Otic Ganglion.
Arnold's Canal; Canal for the auricular branch of the vagus nerve.

Bertin, Exupère, Joseph. 1712-1781
Associate anatomist at the Academy of Sciences, Paris.
Renal Columns – Columnae Bertini.
Sphenoidal Concha – Bones of Bertin. Ligamentum Iliofemorale.

Bigelow, Henry Jacob. 1818-1890.
Professor of surgery at Harvard U.S.A. from 1849-1882
Y-Shaped ligament of Bigelow; The ilio-femoral ligament of the hip-joint, the strongest ligament in the body.

Blumenbach, Johann Friedrich. 1752-1840.
German physiologist and comparative anatomist, becoming professor at Gottingen in 1776.
Blumenbach's bone; Occipital clivis of occipital bone.

Budin, Pierre Constant. 1846-1907
Professor of gynaecology, Paris.
Obstetrical Hinge of Budin.
Joint between the cartilaginous supraoccipital and exoccipital bones.

Chaissaignac, Charles, Marie Edouard 1805-1879.
Professor of anatomy and surgery Paris.
Chaissaignac's Tubercle; Carotid tubercle on the transverse process of the sixth cervical vertebra.

Eustachio, Bartolomeo. 1500-1574.
Professor of anatomy in Rome.
Eustachian Tube; The auditory tube, through which the tympanic cavity communicates with the nasopharynx. The auditory tube was known to Alcmaeon (*fl* 470 B.C.) as long ago as 500 B.C., and Aristole (384-322 B.C.).
Eustachian Valve; Valve of the inferior vena cava.

Fallopio, Gabriele. 1523-1563.
Pupil of Vesalius whom he succeeded in 1551 as professor of anatomy and surgery at Padua.
Fallopian Tubes; Uterine tubes.
Hiatus Fallopio; Hiatus in the greater wing of sphenoid bone for the Greater superficial petrosal nerve.
Fallopian Aquaduct; Facial canal.
He discovered the bony labyrinth in the ear, the auditory, glossopharyngeal and trigmenal nerves and gave the first description of the chorda tympani nerve,, and the Inguinal (Poupart's) ligament in 1584, 121 years before Poupart.

Gasser, Johann Laurentius. 1725-1765
Austrian Professor of Anatomy from 1725 – 1765.
Gasserian Ganglion. Trigeminal Ganglion.

Glaser (Glaserius), Johann Heinrich. 1629-1675.
Professor of Anatomy, Botany and Greek, in Basle.
Fissure of Glaser. Petrotympanic Fissure.

Gido Guida, (Vidius Vidius). 1500-1567.
Vidian Canal; Ptérygoid Canal containing the artery and nerve of the same name

Havers, Clopton. 1657-1702.
In 1698 appointed the first Gale Lecturer at Surgeon's Hall.
Haversian Canal; Vascular canal surrounded by concenteric layers of cortical bone.

Herophilus of Chalcedon. c. 330-260B.C.
A student of Praxagoras of Cos (fl 340 B.C.)
Herophilus is known as the Father of Anatomy. He established the importance of the brain distinguishing, the cerebrum from the cerebellum being the first to grasp the nature of nerves other than those of the special senses. He divided nerves into motor and sensory, describing the meninges and torcular Herophili which still bears his name today. He gave the first description of the lactels which was not improved upon until the publication of the work of Gasparo Aselli (1581-1626) in 1627 posthumously nearly two thousand years later.

Huguier, Pierre Charles. 1804-1873.
Anatomist, Surgeon and Gynaecologist. Paris.
Circle of Huguier, formed at the junction of the cervix and uterus by the uterine arteries.
Sinus of Huguier, a depression in the tympanum between the fenesta ovalis and fenestra rotunda.
Canal of Huguier. Iter Chordae Anterius – Anterior Canaliculus for the Chordae Tympani.

Ingrassia, Giovanni. 1510-1580.
Professor of anatomy Padua.
Processes of Ingrassia; Lesser wings of thesphenoid bone. He is credited with discovering the Auditory tubes in 1546.

Jacobson, Ludwig Levin. 1783-1843.
Anatomist and physician, Copenhagen.
Jacobson's Nerves; Tympanic branch of the glossopharyngeal nerve.
Jacobson's Canal; Canaliculus tympanicus.
Jacobson's Organ; Vomeronasal organ and vomeronasal cartilage.

Lisfranc, de St Martin, Jacques. 1790-1847.
Professor of surgery and operative medicine, Paris.
Lisfranc's Tubercle; Scalene tubercle on the medial border of the first rib.

Lister, Lord Joseph. 1827-1912.
Professor of surgery at Edinburgh 1869, Glasgow 1860 and Kings College Hospital 1877.
Lister's Tubercle; Dorsal radial tubercle of radius.

Louis, Pierre Charles Alexandre. 1787-1872.
Physician in Paris
Angle of Louis; Sternal Angle.

Meckel, Johann Friedrich I the elder. 1714-1774.
Professor of anatomy, botany and gynaecology Berlin.
Meckel's Ganglion; Sphenopalatine ganglion.
Meckel's Cave; Cavum trigeminale containing the trigeminal ganglion.

Meckel, Johann Friedrich II the younger. 1781-1833.
Professor of anatomy and surgery Halle 1808.
Meckel's Cartilage; Cartilage of the 1st branchial arch..
Meckel's Diverticulum; A pouch which projects from the antimesenteric border of the ileum approximately 60cm above the ileo-caecal valve (of Bauhin). In 1700 before Meckel was born, Littre described a hernia containing a Meckel's diverticulum (Littre's Hernia).

Reichert, Karl Bogislaus. 1811-1883.
Professor of human and comparative anatomy Dorpat 1853-83.
Reichert's Cartilage; Cartilage of 2nd branchial arch.
Reichart's Canal; Canal of the deep surface of the transversus abdominus for the passage of the umbilical vein.

Riolan, Jean the Younger. 1580-1657.
Professor of anatomy and botany Paris.
Bones of Riolan; Small ossicles developed along the petro-occipital suture.
Muscle of Riolan; The ciliary bundle, these are very fine fibres found close to the margin of each eyelid, behind the eyelashes.

Scarpa, Antonio. 1747-1832.
Professor of anatomy and surgery Modena 1772, Padua 1783.
Scarpa's Fascia; Deep layer of the superficial fascia of the anterior abdominal wall.
Scarpa's Triangle; Femoral triangle.
Scarpa's Canals; For the palatine branches of the long nasopalatine (Sphenopalatine) nerve, in the incisive fossa.

Sibson, Francis. 1814-1876.
Professor of medicine St Mary's Hospital London.
Sibson's Muscle; Scalenus pleuralis.
Sibson's Fascia; Suprapleural membrane

Stenson, Niels. 1636-1686.
Appointed professor of anatomy in Copenhagen by King Christian V in 1672.
Stensen's Duct; Parotid Duct.
Stensen's Foramen; Sphenopalatine foramen.

Sylvius, Franciscus. 1614-1672.
Professor of practical medicine Leyden 1658.
Aqueduct of Sylvius; Cerebral aqueduct.
Sylvian Fissure; Lateral cerebral fissure.
Sylvian Vein; Superficial middle cerebral vein.

Vesalius, Andreas. 1514-1564.
A pupil of Johannes Günther (1487-1574) of Andernach.
Professor of anatomy Pudua 1535-42.
Foramen of Vesalius; Sphenoidal emissary foramen in the greater wing of sphenoid bone.

Worm, Olas. 1588-1654.
Student of Fabricus at Padua and Bauhin at Basel. In 1624 he succeeded Caspar Bartholin Primus (1585-1620) as professor of anatomy Copenhagen.
Wormian Bones; Small bones found in the sutures of the skull, in particular the Lamboid Suture.

BIBLIOGRAPHY

Bell, J. 1819. Engravings of Bones, Muscles, and Joints. London.

Eustachius, B. 1562. Epistole de Auditus Organis.

Fallopio, G. 1561. Observationes Anatòmicae; P.63.

Gibson. 1716. "Anatomy;" P.489

Santorini, G.D. 1724. Observationes Anatomicae.

Von **Sommering**, T. 1776. De Corpora Humani Fabrica; P.117.

Vesalius, A. 1543. De Corpora Humani Fabrica Basel.

AUTHOR'S NOTE

As a child, Dr David Robson found the human body fascinating. His earliest recollection was discovering a little bird that had fallen from a roof; he remembers dissecting it in order to find the reason it had died.

Since then he has made the study of Anatomy his life's work. His hope is to help others interested in the subject. The idea of the book came about after many students requested that he write such a book.

This is the newest, oldest book on the subject. Enjoy.

And oh! By the way; the autopsy report from a five year old – The bird had died from a broken neck.